THE DEFINITIVE
TESTOSTERONE
REPLACEMENT
THERAPY
MANUAL

HOW TO OPTIMIZE YOUR TESTOSTERONE FOR LIFELONG HEALTH AND HAPPINESS

Written by Jay Campbell

www.TRTRevolution.com

www.FabFitOver40.com

Published by **Archangel Ink**

ISBN: 1942761724
ISBN-13: 978-1-942761-72-3

CONTENTS

About The Definitive Testosterone Replacement Therapy MANual

Jay Campbell has helped thousands of men reclaim their health and masculinity with his Google Hangouts, articles and podcasts on the informed usage of Testosterone Replacement Therapy (also known as TRT).

In *The Definitive Testosterone Replacement Therapy Manual: How to Optimize Your Testosterone for Long term Health and Happiness* you will learn how to:

- Improve your metabolic health
- Increase your mental focus and cognition
- Eliminate feelings of indecisiveness and hesitancy
- Take control of your career while developing more self-confidence at home
- Reinvigorate your sex life and increase the intensity of your libido
- Significantly alter your body composition to one of greater muscle and less body fat
- Ward off the debilitating diseases of aging like diabetes, heart disease and Alzheimer's
- Live a more energetic, empowered and fulfilling life

Men who understand and implement the scientific usage of TRT have dramatically changed their lives for the better by learning how to eliminate the symptoms of low testosterone.

PREFACE

If you are reading this right now you probably have a lot of questions in regards to testosterone and hormone replacement. Just like myself you're probably searching for answers from everything including its effects, how and what it does, how it's used, and every possible pro and con in using a hormone that at its core separates and defines what we are as Men and sets us apart from Women. I once had these questions, I searched the web up and down looking for answers while never being satisfied. That was until I came across Mr. Jay Campbell. After listening to and reading his articles I knew I finally found what I was looking for. A no nonsense, real look, into what exactly hormone replacement therapy is. The more I listened the more intrigued I became.

What I found was a documented diary into someone using hormone replacement as a medical necessity, through a physician, for over a decade, while providing and explaining everything from A-Z. The information was so profound, and moving for me that I eventually reached out to him with other questions and each time Jay would take the time to respond. Today I am very proud to call Jay a close friend.

The knowledge I now possess on hormone replacement and the endocrine system is light years beyond what most, including those in the medical field possess.

Do yourself a favor, and save countless hours of searching like I did. This is the only source you need for understanding what testosterone and hormone replacement therapy is. And how much of a profound effect of how it can have on several aspects of your life. At the very least you will come away with an understanding and the knowledge you need if you choose to take the next step.

-Tony Monticone

WHAT PROGRESSIVE PRACTICING PHYSICIANS SAY ABOUT THE BOOK

Less than 18 months ago I was slaving away, logging hours on the computer as I drafted *GET SERIOUS, A Neurosurgeon's Guide to Optimal Health and Fitness.* Culminated from 30 plus years' experience, its pages touch upon the various risk factors for age-related disease and their modification through practical application of strength training, dietary optimization, stress relief and hormonal therapies. In the context of the latter, the book is lacking in content. I was to a great degree apprehensive about broaching the subject in the wake of the 2013 JAMA study which vilified testosterone therapy. Better stated, I was nervous even though I had a great deal of personal (and overwhelmingly successful) experience with TRT. It was (and still is) an edgy topic. Why? Because there is massive gray area within which lay the overlap between health and ergogenicity or performance enhancement. Conjured are images of Lyle Alzado and Barry Bonds. The stigma of massive men, 'roid rage and now due to the flawed study noted above, coronary artery disease and heart attack. Tons of inertia.

Now close your eyes and erase that deeply-etched slate, if only for a moment. Forget what you've been told and consider only the words of Jay Campbell. Allow him to dispel the many TRT-associated myths while concomitantly describing the myriad benefits in the pages of this book.

A successful real estate agent in the Los Angeles area, Jay is a former physique competitor. He is passionate about health, his darling wife Monica with whom he blogs on <u>FabFitOver40.com</u> and his children. He is dissatisfied with the mean. The word "average" is simply not in his vocabulary. Only optimal is. He is intrigued by the science of performance enhancement, inclusive of both mental and physical aspects, in the context of health. He is not interested in compromising his health to attain the illusion of health as are bodybuilders. That's not what Jay's about. Nor is this book for that matter. This is not another steroid bible. In fact, many of their authors are now ghosts.

In contrast, Jay's goal is longevity. He has come to realize through vast experience that hormonal optimization will stack the biochemical deck in his favor, switching on the genes associated with youth. Testimony to this is his awe-inspiring physique, a side-effect of optimal biochemistry and staunch attention to detail. Inspiring is his knowledge of hormone replacement and human physiology, which surpasses that of many of my medical colleagues. This he brings to you the reader in the pages of his much-needed and timely opus.

So open your eyes, read and digest Jay's words. This book is the chapter that I was scared to write...

Brett Osborn, MD
Diplomate, American Board of Neurological Surgery
Diplomate, American Academy of Anti-Aging Medicine
CSCS, National Strength and Conditioning Association

It is a well-known aphorism that life is a journey. And like so many journeys when we are open minded and aware we stumble upon paths that enlighten us--whether physically, mentally, emotionally, or all of the above. That is what this book is to me--an enlightened path. Not all the readers of this book will look at it in this way and so my foreword may be more about the author, Jay Campbell, then the book itself. For those readers with whom my comments resonate--you will embrace the journey.

I was introduced to Jay about three years ago. We exchanged emails about testosterone replacement therapy and bioidentical hormone treatment. I believe he felt like I was challenging him, coming at him as a mainstream physician. And some part of me was. But Jay was smart, knowledgeable, and resilient. He would come back to me with data. The exchanges became less combative and more cooperative! As my diet and training and nutrition began to evolve, so did my body.

Jay was like a personal trainer pen pal. He helped me direct my extensive medical background, training and dieting experience with his to formulate a comprehensive knowledge base that anyone could benefit from. Hence, this book is the real deal. It gives the reader years of medical research, experience from the gym, and a real world yet scientific understanding of TRT, delivered in a format which WILL HELP anyone wanting to help themselves.

This book is THE resource manual for professionals, strength trainers, athletes and anyone else wanting to utilize Testosterone safely and in the context of health and longevity.

Coming full circle, the book is like furtively reading the journals of countless scientists who have gathered their collective learnings and experiences. For anyone who reads this, they have already begun their journey. The path I stumbled upon when I found Jay Campbell is nothing short of a blessing.

Leonard A. Farber, MD
Clinical Director of Radiation Oncology of Lower Manhattan
Assistant Professor
NY Presbyterian Hospital/Weill Cornell Medical College
The Farber Center for Radiation Oncology

DISCLAIMER

(1) INTRODUCTION

This disclaimer governs the use of this book. [By using this book, you accept this disclaimer in full. We will ask you to agree to this disclaimer before you can access the book.] No part of this book may be reproduced in any written, electronic, recording, or photocopying without written permission of the publisher or authors. All trademarks are the exclusive property of TRTRevolution.com

(2) CREDIT

This disclaimer was created using an SEQ Legal template.

(3) NO ADVICE

The book contains information about Testosterone Replacement Therapy. The information is not advice, and should not be treated as such. You must not rely on the information in the book as an alternative to medical advice from an appropriately qualified professional. If you have any specific questions about any matter you should consult an appropriately qualified medical professional. If you think you may be suffering from any medical condition you should seek immediate medical attention. You should never delay seeking medical advice, disregard medical advice, or discontinue medical treatment because of information in this book

(4) NO REPRESENTATIONS OR WARRANTIES

To the maximum extent permitted by applicable law and subject to section 6 below, we exclude all representations, warranties, undertakings and guarantees relating to the book. Without prejudice to the generality of the foregoing paragraph, we do not represent, warrant, undertake or guarantee:

- that the information in the book is correct, accurate, complete or non-misleading;
- that the use of the guidance in the book will lead to any particular outcome or result;

(5) LIMITATIONS AND EXCLUSIONS OF LIABILITY

The limitations and exclusions of liability set out in this section and elsewhere in this disclaimer: are subject to section 6 below; and govern all liabilities arising under the disclaimer or in relation to the book, including liabilities arising in contract, in tort (including negligence) and for breach of statutory duty. We will not be liable to you in respect of any losses arising out of any event or events beyond our reasonable control. We will not be liable to you in respect of any business losses, including without limitation loss of or damage to profits, income, revenue, use, production, anticipated savings, business, contracts, commercial opportunities or goodwill. We will not be liable to you in respect of any loss or corruption of any data, database or software. We will not be liable to you in respect of any special, indirect or consequential loss or damage.

(6) EXCEPTIONS

Nothing in this disclaimer shall: limit or exclude our liability for death or personal injury resulting from negligence; limit or exclude our liability for fraud or fraudulent misrepresentation; limit any of our liabilities in any way that is not permitted under applicable law; or exclude any of our liabilities that may not be excluded under applicable law.

(7) SEVERABILITY

If a section of this disclaimer is determined by any court or other competent authority to be unlawful and/or unenforceable, the other sections of this disclaimer continue in effect.

If any unlawful and/or unenforceable section would be lawful or enforceable if part of it were deleted, that part will be deemed to be deleted, and the rest of the section will continue in effect.

(8) LAW AND JURISDICTION

This disclaimer will be governed by and construed in accordance with law in the United States of America, and any disputes relating to this disclaimer will be subject to the exclusive jurisdiction of the courts of the United States of America. Testosterone is classified as a controlled substance under the Anabolic Steroids Control Act of 1990 and has been assigned to Schedule III. It is regulated by the Drug Enforcement Agency (DEA).The use of testosterone is illegal in the United States for those without a valid medical diagnosis and prescription justifying their use.

(9) OUR DETAILS

In this disclaimer, "we" means (and "us" and "our" refer to) Jay Campbell (Southern California; USA or any future addresses, temporary or permanent).

ACKNOWLEDGEMENTS

I could not have attempted to write let alone finish this book without the help of the greatest thing that ever happened to me—my unicorn and wife—Monica Diaz. Her enormous power and positive encouragement compelled me to work harder than I ever have before. She taught me the greatest form of acceptance—unyielding and unwavering love and gratitude.

To Jim Brown – my one true mentor who counseled me for years behind the scenes when my doctors were unable. To Dr. Brett Osborn and Dr. Leonard Farber—thanks for being the most scientific gentlemen a guy could know. To Nelson Vergel for being a TRT pioneer and a man with a vision well ahead of its time. To Natalie Minh and Binais Begovic for giving me the forums and advice to platform my knowledge.

To all my family, friends and forum brothers, ex-wives, girlfriends, clients, and fitness industry peers, thank you for the assistance and intel you provided in our times together while researching for more than two decades.

Last but not least, thanks to my dear friend Cary Wan for masterminding this entire process and turning my fragmented intellect into a cogent and enlightening treatise on testosterone replacement therapy.

INTRODUCTION

In the past 25 years, we've been deluged with an endless stream of marketing gimmicks and hyperbolized ad campaigns in newsprint, magazines, television, radio and, most of all, the internet—all designed to sell the latest and greatest "testosterone booster" supplement. To my knowledge, nearly every one of them is a total scam . These products are nothing more than unproven snake oil sold to millions of unsuspecting men who believe and buy into the hype. Men who would do anything to look and feel better. The only thing these supplements have ever done is emptied the bank accounts of those swallowing their "magic pills."

In addition to stopping men from being deceived by the false claims of test booster supplement manufacturers, I wanted to create a definitive resource guide for all men seeking knowledge of legitimate testosterone products, replacement therapy and everything it entails. I had to also consider the greater sociopolitical climate and the controversy surrounding "testosterone" as the taboo and polarizing topic the media has made it out to be.

Whether you are reading this book already convinced of the merits of Testosterone Replacement Therapy (otherwise known as TRT throughout this book), or entirely new to the instrumental role testosterone plays in your life, there is a singular fact that bears repeating; Testosterone is what makes men, MEN. The science of this is indisputable. Testosterone, when administered properly and in clinical dose fashion, has the potential to revitalize male life across every conceivable aspect of health. Whether it be increased musculature, improved metabolic health, or the improved cognitive and psychologic benefits, testosterone CAN BE your "silver bullet."

If you are one of the fortunate who has already sought out TRT and experienced its many benefits, this book will educate you to the bleeding edge of TRT science and strategy. It will be your bible for making the most informed decision possible when working with a progressive TRT physician and/or designing your own customized TRT therapy.

Or, you may be one of the millions whose natural testosterone levels have declined so dramatically that your "zest" for life no longer exists. Whether you're in your 30s or younger, or even approaching "middle age," deep inside, you question whether it is your destiny to endure feeling this lousy.

My book is proof positive your life does not have to be this way. Not only can it be avoided, it can be made nonexistent through the transformative power of testosterone replacement therapy. I encourage you to read on to understand how TRT can be your paradigm-changing solution for living an exciting and purposeful life.

Is There a War on Men?

WAR ON MEN

The truth about testosterone is hard to find. Although we supposedly live in an era when scientific inquiry thrives, many remain ignorant about the single most important hormone in the male body. If Aristotle were around, he would call this hormone the *sine qua non* of masculinity. Without this hormone, you are not a man. Indeed, transgender women who want to transition into men inject this drug. It is the hormone responsible for normal growth and development of male sex characteristics.

Testosterone formulations were partially synthesized from a cholesterol base by Adolf Butenandt at Schering in 1935[1]. For his work, he was awarded the Nobel Prize in Chemistry, which he shared with another steroid chemist, Leopold Ruzicka in 1939[2]. Both testosterone and its derivatives quickly became the target of invention and application to both humans and animals during the golden age of testosterone chemistry (from 1950 to the mid-1960's), with the development of 'testosterone esters'[3]. These were chemical compounds designed to

---

1   Szöllösi-Janze, Margit (2001). Science in the Third Reich (German Historical Perspectives). Oxford, UK: Berg Publishers. ISBN 1-85973-421-9.

2   Karl Grandin, ed. (1939). "Leopold Ružička Biography". Les Prix Nobel. The Nobel Foundation. Retrieved 2008-10-21

3   Schwarz S, Onken D, Schubert A (July 1999). "The steroid story of Jenapharm: from the late 1940s to the early 1970s". Steroids 64 (7): 439–45.

slow down the breakdown of testosterone in the human body. Using testosterone esters allowed physicians to harness these powerful tissue-building drugs to better study and effectively treat a variety of medical conditions, including hypogonadism, anemia, wasting diseases, burns, recovery from surgery and trauma, age-related frailty, and many others.

Most professional bodybuilders, fitness competitors, pro athletes, celebrity actors, and political leaders who use testosterone are forced to conceal their use. They must pretend to be 100% natural, both to maintain their image and because the U.S. government classifies non-prescription testosterone use as a felony crime. The media won't tell you the truth about TRT because the media is waging a war against testosterone[4]. Regardless of why, the reality is testosterone levels in men are dramatically decreasing and have been for more than 20 years across the USA[5].

It is imperative you attempt to consult with a doctor who knows what he or she is doing when prescribing TRT. Unfortunately, this eliminates a huge percentage of physicians.[6] This book is not meant as a backhanded slight to the established medical community who otherwise attempt to offer help by prescribing wide-ranging protocols of TRT to their patients. Many are doing the best they can with limited information and long-term studies available to them.

This book is one of the first of its kind to attempt to create a better resource for TRT-prescribing physicians and their patients. It offers the hard-earned wisdom and calculated advice of men who have used TRT productively for more than a decade under the aid and clinical supervision of experienced and forward-thinking doctors. This advice is backed by highly relevant scientific research, citation and data to clearly substantiate truth from widely held myths and misbeliefs.

My book displays an unbridled passion for molecular biology, biochemistry and endocrinology, but is written for all men to easily understand. A book that dispels all the TRT misnomers and

---

4   http://www.nytimes.com/2014/09/18/health/testosterone-drugs-fda.html

5   A population-level decline in serum testosterone levels in American men. J Clin Endocrinol Metab. 2007 Jan;92(1):196-202. Epub 2006 Oct 24.

6   Are We Testing Appropriately for Low Testosterone?: Characterization of Tested Men and Compliance with Current Guidelines. Malik RD1, Lapin B, Wang CE, Lakeman JC, Helfand BT. J Sex Med. 2014 Nov 10. doi:

conventional beliefs held by far too many men for too long. A book which offers scientific yet practical TRT information no aging man should be without.

No one person or corporation owns the author of this book. I can and will tell you the truth about testosterone. Are you ready to learn how TRT can improve your life in every conceivable fashion?

This is not a book about Anabolic Steroids. There have been plenty of authoritative books written by superb researchers and scientists about using Anabolics[7],[8]. This book is a resource guide written for men on how to use testosterone productively for life. It provides crystal-clear strategies designed to optimize physical and mental performance while enjoying the benefits of TRT. There is a difference between testosterone use versus abuse[9].

7   Roberts Anthony, Clapp Brian-Anabolic Steroids Ultimate Research Guide Volume 1. 2005 Anabolic Information LLC. www.anabolicbooks.com

8   William Llewellyn, Anabolics 10th Edition. 2010 Molecular Nutrition.

9   http://www.defymedical.com/resources/105

Becoming an Empowered Man through Optimal Blood Testosterone Levels: The Physical Benefits

Chapter 2

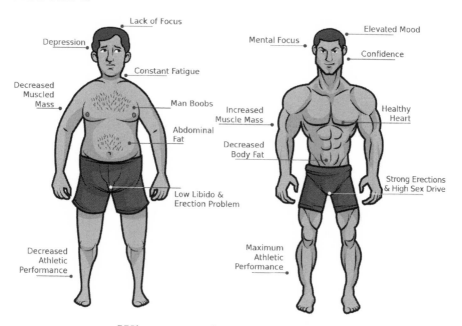

Why men need more testosterone

My mission in writing this book is helping to create powerful, driven, confident men who want the most out of their lives. By raising your testosterone level to the highest end of the optimal range through legitimately prescribed testosterone, you'll ensure your life is enhanced in almost every capacity imaginable. This book will analyze and dissect the various accepted TRT protocols to provide you with the latest and most cutting-edge research available. I will also point out the pros and cons of choosing the counsel and aid of a TRT-prescribing doctor while also working with them via the route of self-administration (when approved and instructed by your prescribing physician).

When people ask why they should consider having their testosterone measured, the only answer worthy of the question is "to understand if you're functioning optimally as a man." Although controversy remains regarding indications for testosterone supplementation in men due to a lack of large-scale, long-term studies assessing the benefits and risks of TRT, reports from thousands of men and their doctors prescribing TRT indicate it often produces a wide range of benefits. In fact testosterone usage has never been significantly widespread, as the number of patients with a testosterone prescription rose from 1.3 million people in 2010 to 2.3 million in 2013[10]. These numbers are obviously not reflective of the global male population base using TRT without a prescription. It's estimated there are about 6 million people[11] (without a prescription) using anabolic and/or androgenic steroids (including testosterone) or human growth hormone (HGH) every year.

According to the U.S. Census Bureau, approximately 15 million men have low testosterone levels also known as Andropause[12]. Shockingly, only 5% to 10% of these men will seek treatment. 'Male hypogonadism' as it's also known is a recognized medical condition which remains underdiagnosed by many doctors.

Hypogonadism is often underdiagnosed for the following reasons:

1. Men don't report it to their doctors because they are embarrassed due to their symptoms being sexual in nature. Additionally, they are conditioned to accept these symptoms as being a typical result of 'old age' and thus uncorrectable.

---

10   Will the FDA Tighten the Use of Testosterone Replacement Therapy? http://www.hcplive.com/medical-news/will-the-fda-tighten-the-use-of-testosterone-replacement-therapy
11   http://www.criminaldefenselawyer.com/resources/illegal-steroids-and-human-growth-hormone-hgh.htm
12   Andropause: Current concepts .Indian J Endocrinol Metab. 2013 Dec;17(Suppl 3):S621-9. doi: 10.4103/2230-8210.123552

2. Men present with nonspecific symptoms such as lack of motivation, depression, listlessness, etc. Rarely is low testosterone suspected as the source for these symptoms.
3. There isn't a definitive biochemical test for hypogonadism.
4. There is a distinct lack of physician awareness of the condition. Many doctors do not understand what blood tests to order and how to effectively identify the symptoms of a testosterone deficiency.

I believe the estimated number of 15 million men with symptoms of low T is drastically underestimated. There are men seemingly everywhere who dress, walk, and talk effeminately. It is now commonplace to see men who are riddled with estrogenic fat deposition. To say it is an underdiagnosed problem would be an understatement.

Any man reading this book should find comfort in the reams of recent scientific and anecdotal data espousing the benefits of TRT. But more importantly you should feel supremely confident you are following the advice of those who have mastered the art of TRT from every level of physical and mental significance. Men who now live with benefits so numerous and life-enhancing it is imperative to give those contemplating TRT a clearer picture of what to expect.

TESTOSTERONE DECREASES BODY FAT

Testosterone is essential to the regulation of insulin, glucose, and fat storage.[13] As testosterone levels plummet, so does your body's ability to process the insulin, glucose, and fat. Simply put, a decrease in T levels is directly correlated with an increase in fat storage.[14]

To make matters worse for obese men, an increase in fat also lowers T levels. The fatter you become the lower your testosterone. This brutal cycle is a huge contributor to the obesity pandemic sweeping the world. In obese males there is increased aromatase activity, which irreversibly converts testosterone to estradiol, resulting in decreased testosterone and elevated estrogen levels. However, obese and high body fat men alike can break this cycle by undergoing TRT, as testosterone is lipolytic[15] (i.e. fat burning). Studies have also shown that one of the positive benefits of testosterone treatment is a decrease in adiposity also known as fat storage.[16] I discuss the role of testosterone, aromatase, and obesity much more in Chapter 9.

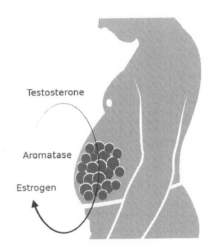

13   The interactions between hypothalamic-pituitary-adrenal axis activity, testosterone, insulin-like growth factor I and abdominal obesity with metabolism and blood pressure in men.Int J Obes Relat Metab Disord. 1998 Dec;22(12):1184-96.

14   Obesity in men: The hypogonadal–estrogen receptor relationship and its effect on glucose homeostasis Cohen, Paul G.Medical Hypotheses , Volume 70 , Issue 2 , 358 – 360

15   Høst C, Gormsen LC, Christensen B, et al. Independent Effects of Testosterone on Lipid Oxidation and VLDL-TG Production: A Randomized, Double-Blind, Placebo-Controlled, Crossover Study. Diabetes 2013;62(5):1409-1416. doi:10.2337/db12-0440.

16   Predictors of skeletal muscle mass in elderly men and women. Mech Ageing Dev. 1999;107:123–136. [PubMed]

TESTOSTERONE INCREASES MUSCLE MASS

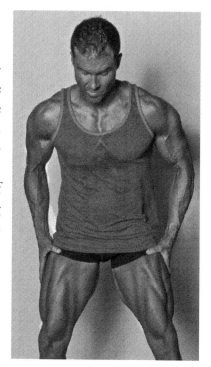

Testosterone is an essential muscle-building hormone. Testosterone is the basis of muscle, of strength, and the source of what makes men powerful. Testosterone builds muscle by increasing muscle protein synthesis.[17]

What does that mean? It means if you exercise with weights while using testosterone you'll build larger muscles and increase your overall strength.

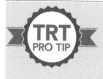

It is important to understand that a clean diet and a sound resistance training program are absolutely necessary to maximize the potential benefits of TRT.[18] I discuss this much more in Chapters 11 and 12.

---

17   132. Verhaar HJJ, Samson MM, Aleman A, de Vries WR, de Vreede PL, Koppeschaar HPF. The relationship between indices of muscle function and circulating anabolic hormones in healthy.Aging Male. 2000;3:75–80

18   Effects of progressive resistance training on growth hormone and testosterone levels in young and elderly subjects. Craig BW, Brown R, Everhart J.Mech Ageing Dev. 1989 Aug; 49(2):159-69.

TESTOSTERONE IMPROVES HEART HEALTH

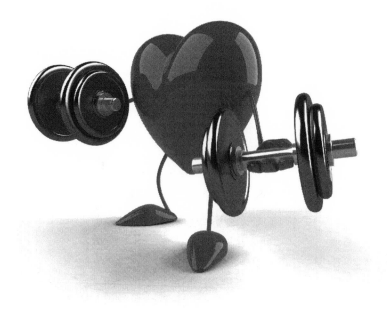

Until very recently, researchers have been divided on the topic of how testosterone affects heart health. Some researchers have claimed high T levels are linked to heart disease while others have found low T is responsible for an increased risk of heart ailments.[19] Ultimately, there is convincing evidence[20] maintaining superlative T levels can help prevent cardiovascular disease.[21] "Help" is the keyword here. The benefits that come with healthy testosterone levels, not testosterone alone, are what allows the heart to maintain its strength. I offer much more information about testosterone and its effect on the heart and vascular networks later in Chapter 9.

---

19   Prevention of coronary artery disease in men: Male hormone, female hormone, or both? Yang, Changsheng et al. Medical Hypotheses , Volume 75 , Issue 6 , 671 – 673

20   http://www.webmd.com/men/news/20140702/latest-study-finds-no-link-between-testosterone-supplements-heart-attack

21   Testosterone as an atrial fibrillation treatment and stroke preventative in aging men: Case histories and hypothesis Eby, George Medical Hypotheses , Volume 75 , Issue 2 , 269 – 270

 The hyperbolic fear about testosterone replacement therapy causing increased CVD (cardiovascular disease)[22] events in otherwise normal and healthy men is unsupported. There is little data or proof substantiating the national TV, newsprint, and internet ads you've likely seen from legal groups and attorneys claiming TRT increases the risk of heart attacks, stroke, CVD, etc. Absurdly, the foundational study that prompted this CVD risk witch hunt came from a clinical trial (TOM trial) investigating the use of a topical TRT in men over 65 with limited mobility—men who could barely walk or move on their own[23]. The preponderance of evidence clearly indicates an increased risk of cardiovascular disease and death in general, in men with low or low normal testosterone blood levels[24]. TRT when dosed and maintained to optimal levels offers no increased risk of CVD and may in fact offer CVD protection. Later in Chapter 10 and also in the interview with Dr. Brett Osborn in Chapter 13, I will back up this assertion with the most relevant and recent research data.

22   http://www.trtrev.com/wp-content/uploads/2015/10/Testosterone-Therapy-and-Cardiovascular-Risk.pdf

23   Basaria S, Davda MN, Travison TG, Ulloor J, Singh R, Bhasin S. Risk Factors Associated With Cardiovascular Events During Testosterone Administration in Older Men With Mobility Limitation. The Journals of Gerontology Series A: Biological Sciences and Medical Sciences. 2013;68(2):153-160. doi:10.1093/gerona/gls 138.

24   Xu L, Freeman G, Cowling BJ, Schooling CM. Testosterone therapy and cardiovascular events among men: a systematic review and meta-analysis of placebo-controlled randomized trials. BMC Medicine 2013;11:108. doi:10.1186/1741-7015-11-108.

TESTOSTERONE INCREASES BONE DENSITY

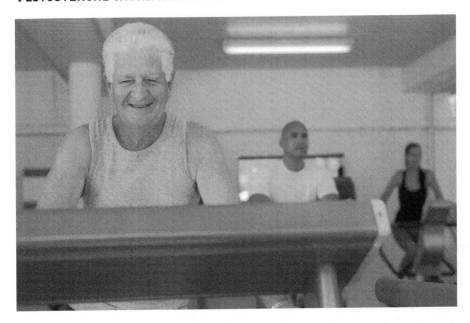

Men can be at risk of bone diseases as well, and low testosterone is surely a causative factor. Testosterone is indisputably linked to bone health.[25] It increases bone density and impedes the bone resorption that comes with age[26].

It has been noted that men who suffer from bone disease usually have low testosterone.[27] The last thing any man wants is to end up with a deteriorated hip or spine—completely limiting their movement and range of motion in later life.

If you want ideal bone health into your later years, you owe it to yourself to improve your testosterone levels.

---

25   Selective estrogen receptor modulators: A possible new treatment of osteoporosis in males
Kastelan, Darko et al. Medical Hypotheses , Volume 67 , Issue 5 , 1052 – 1053
26   Male osteoporosis: clinical approach and management in family practice.Singapore Med J. 2014 Jul;55(7):353-7.
27   Fink HA, Ewing SK, Ensrud KE, et al. Association of testosterone and estradiol deficiency with osteoporosis and rapid bone loss in older men. J Clin Endocrinol Metab. 2006;91(10):3908–39015.[PubMed]

TESTOSTERONE COMBATS ALZHEIMER'S DISEASE AND IMPROVES COGNITION

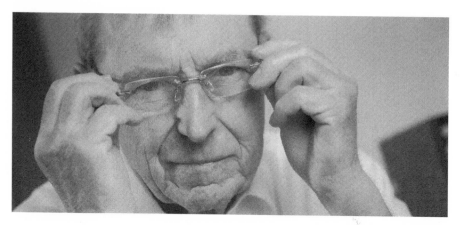

Studies show many older men with mild cognitive issues suffer from low testosterone.[28] Many of these men eventually develop Alzheimer's.[29] At the University of Southern California, researchers noted that increasing T levels in older men stalled the development of Alzheimer's. This has led scientists to speculate maintaining healthy testosterone levels may actually prevent Alzheimer's[30]. There is clear and substantial evidence TRT improves memory as men age.[31] If you are an aging man and interested in preserving your memory well into your golden years, it's a very good preventative measure to ensure your testosterone levels are optimized.

28   Gillett MJ, Martins RN, Clarnette RM, Chubb SA, Bruce DG, Yeap BB. Relationship between testosterone, sex hormone binding globulin and plasma amyloid beta peptide 40 in older men with subjective memory loss or dementia. J Alzheimers Dis. 2003;5:267–269. [PubMed]

29   Plasma testosterone levels in Alzheimer and Parkinson diseases. Okun MS, DeLong MR, Hanfelt J, Gearing M, Levey A. Neurology. 2004 Feb 10;62(3):411-3.

30   Cunningham RL, Singh M, O'Bryant SE, Hall JR, Barber RC. Oxidative stress, testosterone, and cognition among Caucasian and Mexican American men with and without Alzheimer's disease. Journal of Alzheimer's disease : JAD. 2014;40(3):563-573. doi:10.3233/JAD-131994.

31   Can testosterone replacement decrease the memory problem of old age? Lim, David et al.Medical Hypotheses , Volume 60 , Issue 6 , 893 – 896

Testosterone and A Fulfilled Life

Chapter 3

Testosterone Will Improve Your Confidence with Sexual

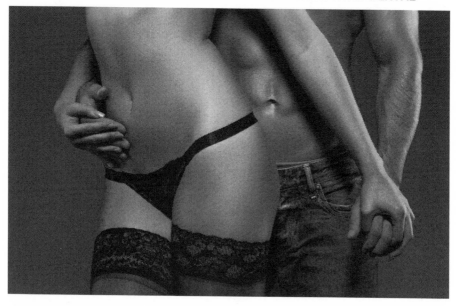

Partners

In the animal world, high testosterone levels have been shown to be linked to dominance in the battle for mates. The same is true for humans. Studies have shown when two men were instructed to vie for the affections of a woman, the man's aggression, ability to direct the interaction, and chances of attracting the woman were associated with their testosterone levels before the task.[32] So there is truth in the idea

---

32   Sex-hormone dependent perception of androstenone suggests its involvement in communicating competition and aggression. Lübke KT1, Pause BM. Physiol Behav. 2014 Jan 17;123:136-41. doi: 10.1016/j.physbeh.2013.10.016. Epub 2013 Oct 25

that boldness is a powerful key to attracting potential mates. There is little doubt testosterone is responsible for this boldness.

Improving your testosterone level can increase your ability to approach suitors and build quick rapport. From an evolutionary biology standpoint, women sense and are attracted to higher testosterone in men and enjoy communication with males who give off an aura of high T.[33] There is even research[34] indicating women smell higher testosterone and seek it out during various points of their menstrual cycle. Knowing this, if you struggle with approaching women or dating, why would you not want to investigate the route of testosterone replacement therapy (TRT)?

MORE TESTOSTERONE EQUALS HEIGHTENED SEX DRIVE AND LIBIDO

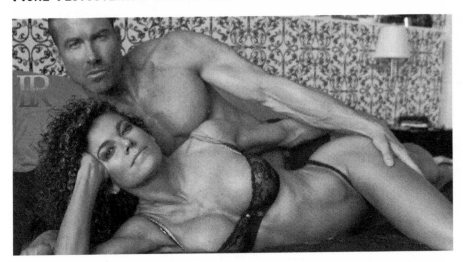

There's an entire industry devoted to correcting low libido and erectile dysfunction through artificial chemicals. Supplementing with TRT can dramatically increase sex drive and improve the quality and quantity of erections.[35] Testosterone is the most powerful male

33   Sex-hormone dependent perception of androstenone suggests its involvement in communicating competition and aggression. Lübke KT1, Pause BM. Physiol Behav. 2014 Jan 17;123:136-41. doi: 10.1016/j.physbeh.2013.10.016. Epub 2013 Oct 25

34   http://www.huffingtonpost.com/2013/04/18/mens-smell-testosterone-attractive-to-women-study_n_3110182.html

35   145. Wang C, Cunningham G, Dobs A, et al. Long-term testosterone gel (Andro-Gel) treatment maintains beneficial effects on sexual function and mood, lean and fat mass,

sex hormone, and many male sexual issues can be reversed through a testosterone improvement regimen.

Unfortunately, many men who otherwise suffer from low Testosterone, are routinely scripted Viagra or Cialis and an anti-depressant when they present to their doctor with a lowered libido. Astute TRT physicians need to learn how to decipher whether a patient has a lack of desire or a real life inability to perform (low T). As will be stated continually in this book – symptoms and then blood panels MUST be taken into account before cavalierly dispensing erectile dysfunction and mood altering medications.

TESTOSTERONE WILL IMPROVE YOUR MINDSET

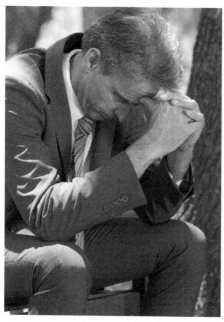

Many men today are buried under the dark soil of depression and it is abundantly clear that low testosterone levels are to blame.[36] Sadly, scientists are stuck trying to figure out a biological riddle akin to the chicken or the egg: does low testosterone cause depression, or does depression cause low testosterone? Despite this confusion, research demonstrates that men undergoing testosterone treatments have reported improvements in mood and other issues related to depression.[37] Many of these same men have overwhelmingly improved

and bone mineral density in hypogonadal men. J Clin Endocrinol Metab. 2004;89:2085–2098. [PubMed]

36   The role of sex and sex-related hormones in cognition, mood and well-being in older men and women.
Biol Psychol. 2014 Sep 6;103C:158-166. doi: 10.1016/j.biopsycho.2014.08.015. [Epub ahead of prin

37   The effects of pharmacologically induced hypogonadism on mood in healthy men.
Arch Gen Psychiatry. 2004;61:997–1004. [PubMed] 147. Schmidt PJ, Berlin KL, Danaceau MA, et al.

their psychological capacity, giving them a feeling of reclaiming their life. In fact, the brain fog exhibited by men suffering from testosterone deficiency, is often eliminated completely upon implementing an intelligent TRT protocol. The fastest noticeable positive effects of TRT is clearer thinking and an improved mood.

THE COMPETITIVE EDGE FROM TESTOSTERONE

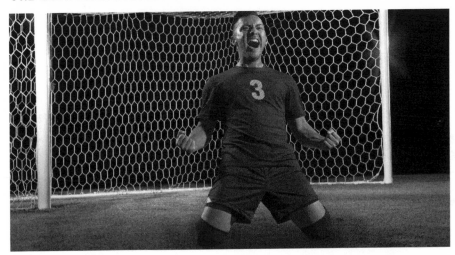

Testosterone is responsible for the masculine need for victory and challenge.[38] It also greatly speeds up reaction times, improves eyesight and endurance and produces feelings of invulnerability.[39]

In fact, one study shows a man's testosterone levels are predictive of whether he will persevere through defeat or give in when faced with a challenge.[40]

---

38   Intercollegiate soccer: saliva cortisol and testosterone are elevated during competition, and testosterone is related to status and social connectedness with team mates. Edwards DA1, Wetzel K, Wyner DR PLoS One. 2012;7(4):e34814. doi: 10.1371/journal.pone.0034814. Epub 2012 Apr 18.

39   Serum testosterone, growth hormone, and insulin-like growth factor-1 levels, mental reaction time, and maximal aerobic exercise in sedentary and long-term physically trained elderly males. Int J Neurosci. 2004 May;114(5):623-37.

40   Implicit power motivation predicts men's testosterone changes and implicit learning in a contest situation. Schultheiss OC1, Rohde W. Horm Behav. 2002 Mar;41(2):195-202.

Think of the times in your life when you've experienced the "thrill of victory" when one of the sports teams you watched or played on won a big game. It's quite exhilarating. The same might be felt in the business world when achieving a big sale or finalizing a huge deal. There is documented scientific evidence showing testosterone increases exponentially for days in men after winning a game or achieving a great feat.[41] Imagine having those feelings as a part of your day-to-day life when using TRT.

TAKE RISKS, ACHIEVE STATUS

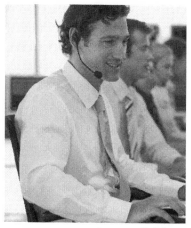

Testosterone has been linked to risk-taking and higher status in men. Men with high testosterone and high status tend to be more risk-averse than their low testosterone, low status brethren. Studies indicate this is because these men have more to hold onto than their low status brothers, as evidenced by the benefits summarized above.

Interestingly, testosterone levels are noted to increase after every victory a person experiences.[42] This trend of increases creates a positive loop where the high testosterone victor may triumph over an opponent with more skill but less testosterone.

---

41   Testosterone and cortisol release among Spanish soccer fans watching the 2010 World Cup final. van der Meij L1, Almela M, Hidalgo V, Villada C, Ijzerman H, van Lange PA, Salvador A

42   Changes in testosterone mediate the effect of winning on subsequent aggressive behaviour.
Carré JM1, Campbell JA, Lozoya E, Goetz SM, Welker KM. Psychoneuroendocrinology. 2013 Oct;38(10):2034-41. doi: 10.1016/j.psyneuen.2013.03.008. Epub 2013 Apr 12.

OPTIMAL TESTOSTERONE, YOUR MOST POWERFUL AND ENLIGHTENED SELF

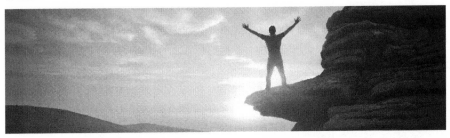

When you have higher levels of testosterone your ability to be ultra-confident in your decisions and take decisive action is exponentially increased. You are assertive and purposeful in all that you do and say. Your decisions empower you to behave in ways others find attractive.

Supplementing with testosterone will help a beta-male become more assertive giving him more alpha like characteristics. It will make an alpha male more focused, determined and a leader among his peers.

There are many people who espouse theories on raising testosterone naturally.

While it's true tweaking your diet and nutritional supplement protocol to optimize your testosterone can offer some help as can certain posture improvement exercises, nothing is as powerful or universally proven as using pharmaceutical TRT. Especially utilizing one of the TRT protocols recommended in the pages of this book.

The Science of Testosterone 101: Why Men MUST Understand Their Endocrinology

Chapter 4

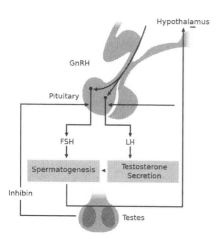

Hormonal Control of Testosterone

What is Testosterone and How is It Made?

Testosterone is a hormone both males and females need in the right amount to function properly, not only physically but mentally. Our focus is on men who don't want to live within what is defined as the "normal range" of testosterone. Even more important is preventing men from experiencing the symptoms of low testosterone. It is not the purpose of this book to offer a deep analysis of the male endocrine and reproductive system. We will offer a quick and simple explanation of what testosterone is and how it works in men.

Testosterone plays many different roles as we age. In early development it is vital for brain, sex, and bone formation. Later in life, it's important for brain chemistry, maintaining muscle mass, and sexual function.[43] Your body has regulation systems in place to keep things operational. For example if you eat sugar, your body has chemical receptors that pick up the increase of glucose in your bloodstream and

---

43   Mooradian AD, Morley JE, Korenman SG (February 1987). "Biological actions of androgens". Endocr. Rev. 8 (1): 1–28. doi:10.1210/edrv-8-1-1. PMID 3549275.

in response release insulin to regulate your blood sugar and maintain homeostasis. The same happens with testosterone production.

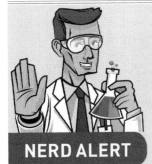

NERD ALERT

Your brain will send a chemical sign to the hypothalamus saying it needs some testosterone made. The hypothalamus will in turn release a messenger called gonadotropin (GnRH) that is picked up by the pituitary gland. This causes the pituitary gland to release luteinizing hormone (LH) and follicle-stimulating hormone (FSH). These will be recognized by the Leydig cells in the testes to synthesize testosterone. The testosterone is then released where it will be bound to sex hormone-binding globulin (SHBG) and albumin or will remain in its free form and in turn find targeted cells to bind with.

There is a negative feedback loop known as the Hypothalamic-Pituitary-Testicular-Axis (HPTA) also now known as the hypothalamic–pituitary–gonadal axis (HPGA) that will send messages to the pituitary saying there is enough testosterone in the system. The pituitary will in turn slow production of LH and eventually FSH. Testosterone will be reduced into a number of other metabolites that serve important functions such as dihydrotestosterone (DHT) or estradiol (E2). I will discuss these in much more depth later in the book in Chapter 10.

WHY DO YOU STOP PRODUCING OPTIMAL LEVELS OF T?

As we age our body isn't as efficient with maintaining proper testosterone production and our homeostasis level is set too low. This could be in response to an injury such as damaged testes. Blunt trauma (a strike)[44] accounts for 75% of testicular injuries. These can occur from getting kicked, hit by a baseball, motorcycle/bicycle accident, etc.

The honest truth which few others have the courage to write about is our horrific environmental situation. All around the world men's endocrine systems are being bombarded[45] via the increase in environmental pollutants, contaminants and particulates in the air produced by industrial factories, smog and emissions from cars, etc.

44   http://www.webmd.com/men/guide/testicle-injuries

45   http://www.ewg.org/research/dirty-dozen-list-endocrine-disruptors

Men are under siege from hormonal suppressing phytoestrogens[46] (such as soy protein by-products[47]), and a host of other toxins as a direct result of modern day societal living.

Exposure to *phthalates*, which are found in many plastics is "feminizing" boys by blocking normal male testosterone.[48] Even men's sperm counts are falling due to exposure to pesticides, endocrine-disrupting chemicals like bisphenol A (BPA)[49], and the many other toxins increasingly pervading our water and food supplies. Phthalates are now a horrific modern day problem for not only men, but also women and children. There is now animal and human evidence that exposure to phthalates (chemicals found in plastics and personal care products) is associated with reduced androgen levels and associated disorders.[50]

Regardless of the cause, when this happens you will eventually have such low levels of testosterone you'll start to feel differently, both mentally and physically over time. And before you know it, you'll feel "old" and nothing like you used to when you were "young".

Once a man has reached this low level of testosterone and if fortunate enough to be diagnosed by a physician, he is classified as being hypogonadal. The most recent accepted data is half of all men over the age of fifty are classified as hypogonadal. As I have already stated, it is clear from societal observation this number is significantly underestimated. For the purposes of keeping it simple to understand, there are two forms of diagnosed hypogonadism:

---

46   Are oestrogens involved in falling sperm counts and disorders of the male reproductive tract?". Lancet 341 (8857): 1392–5.doi:10.1016/0140-6736 Sharpe RM, Skakkebaek NE (1993).

47   http://fabfitover40.com/2014/06/06/soy-protein-friend-foe/

48   How dangerous are phthalate plasticizers? Integrated approach to toxicity based on metabolism, electron transfer, reactive oxygen species and cell signaling Kovacic, Peter Medical Hypotheses , Volume 74 , Issue 4 , 626 – 628

49   How safe is bisphenol A? Fundamentals of toxicity: Metabolism, electron transfer and oxidative stress
Kovacic, Peter Medical Hypotheses , Volume 75 , Issue 1 , 1 – 4

50   Urinary phthalate metabolites are associated with decreased serum testosterone in men, women, and children from NHANES 2011-2012. J Clin Endocrinol Metab. 2014 Nov;99(11):4346-52. doi: 10.1210/jc.2014-2555. Epub 2014 Aug 14.

Primary Hypogonadism results from defects of the gonads. Luteinizing hormone (LH) and/or follicle stimulating hormone (FSH) are usually elevated, meaning the problem is in the testicles.

Secondary Hypogonadism results from hypothalamic or pituitary defects. Luteinizing hormone (LH) and/or follicle stimulating hormone (FSH) are normal or low, suggesting the problem is in the brain, i.e. a disruption in the HTPA/HPGA.

Many doctors classify 'normal aging' as the cause of secondary hypogonadism. This author refuses to accept getting softer, weaker, depressed and having a low libido as 'normal' and healthy aging. Why would you or any man you know for that matter want to feel this way? Especially knowing there was a way to keep your testosterone elevated to optimal levels for life through the intelligent and scientific usage of TRT.

How Do I Know I Need TRT?

Chapter 5

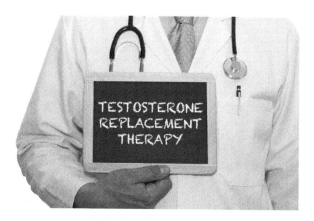

As a voracious researcher of the most recent and relevant medical studies, while at the same time utilizing TRT for more than a decade under close Doctor supervision, I've come to realize there are crucial factors necessary to consider when making the decision to proceed with TRT.

The Ethical Dilemma of Testosterone-Pick Your Side

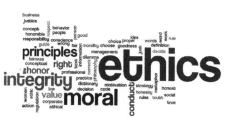

One of the biggest challenges men face is overcoming any moral qualms they have before undergoing TRT. It is my duty to explain there is absolutely nothing morally wrong with restoring your testosterone levels back to "above normal" levels or better. Testosterone is a naturally occurring hormone in both the male and female endocrine system. The fact that a naturally occurring hormone, essential to the development of every human being on planet Earth, is controlled and demonized – is absurd. But this is the paradigm we find ourselves in.

As a sovereign adult male, it is your responsibility to turn lemons into lemonade.

There are no limits to the factors working AGAINST you— stress, diet, pollution, age, popular culture, etc. If you don't stand up for yourself, who else will? This is a silent pandemic. The vast majority of men aren't even aware low testosterone is an issue. Your friends and family, and likely even yourself, have been conditioned through the mass media to believe "using testosterone is cheating", "drugs are bad" and "getting old is just an accepted part of life".

While this book is not meant to be a treatise disputing the current war on drugs – let me put it to you this way:

- If you had a headache, would you swallow an Aspirin tablet so you can stop your head from pounding?
- If you have High Cholesterol and need Lipitor, would you take the drug to reduce your cardio-vascular risk factors?
- If you have unbearable pain and can only get around in a wheelchair for the rest of your life unless you got a hip replacement, would you allow a surgeon to replace your joints so you can walk again?

If you answered "yes" to any of these questions, then please understand the morality is no different when restoring the hormone that best defines your masculinity. It's just like waking up in the morning and making a cup of coffee so you can start your day with a little caffeine. TRT is a scientifically proven and acceptable treatment. While it has not yet gained widespread social acceptance, remember great men never follow the herd. You owe it to yourself to consider the program outlined in this book.

TESTOSTERONE DECLINES WITH AGE

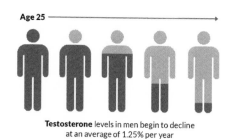

Age 25

Testosterone levels in men begin to decline at an average of 1.25% per year

This is a difficult factor to tackle especially in light of the "Beta Male Syndrome[51]" many young men in their late teens and early 20's are experiencing today. Ten years ago, I generally would have recommended TRT no sooner than 35 years old but it's becoming more and more apparent low testosterone is a significant problem in men of all ages—especially younger ones.

For *any man under the age of 30 with symptoms of low T,* you must find a doctor willing to measure your blood panels and selectively examine your presenting symptoms. Especially if your testosterone is proven to be low or low-normal. Any young man below the age of 30 wanting to embark on a course of TRT should do their homework. I have written this book as a step-by-step guide for men of all ages but I'd be a fool to not tell much younger men to proceed cautiously and learn as much as possible before embarking down the path of TRT.

TRT PRO TIP The younger you are and especially if your goal is to father children, your doctor should FIRST consider alleviating the stressor or cause of your hypogonadal state. This is preferable to placing a drug in your body (T) which can seize control and or shut down your endocrine system (your body's natural production of testosterone). If this fails, the next step would be prescribing medications that attempt to raise T (which are not disruptive (or minimally so) of your body's natural production of testosterone. These medications are written about in depth later in the book in Chapters 9 and 10.

---

51   http://www.dangerandplay.com/2014/05/24/meeting-dp-readers-shocked/

 It is important to understand utilizing TRT productively (in whichever delivery system is best for you) is a lifelong strategy. Financial stability is a necessity as engaging in TRT is not without costs. Being able to pay for your treatment and also ancillary medications (when necessary) must be factored into day-to-day life expenses. Hence, it is hard for me to recommend TRT for early 20 something's men who are unlikely financially stable (this is assuming your blood test and presenting symptoms qualify you for a doctor's prescription of TRT).

It is also an unfortunate fact many physicians will frown upon younger men (under the age of 35) who desire to proceed down the path of TRT. You must respect your doctor's desire for discretion as there have been legal issues for doctors who prescribed testosterone for what was perceived to be 'outside the bounds of medical usage.' If you do choose this course of action, be prepared to intelligently discuss your options with an informed TRT physician based on your symptoms first, blood work second. And make absolutely sure you will be able to afford it. Most importantly, make sure your doctor pursues less disruptive forms or testosterone restoration first (eliminating stressors and using either hCG or clomid monotherapy).

I have many anecdotal stories from young men who enjoy the hefty benefits of TRT in their work life (becoming assertive on the job, closing more sales, getting promotions). These men can't imagine going back to their normal "pre-T" lives. They have fit TRT into their monthly budget as a critical investment into their personal and professional development. In a nutshell, they make more money at work and in business while on TRT to justify the costs many times over.

If you are a much younger man who feels you are suffering from the symptoms of low T and would benefit from TRT, I recommend you first go online and pay for an independent assay to see if your testosterone blood levels are at a level low enough for you to seek out an experienced TRT Doctor and initiate a conversation. You can do that by going to this website: http://TRTRev.com/blood-tests

But remember: *low testosterone is a clinical as opposed to a laboratory diagnosis*. It is not simply "low testosterone" on blood testing. What constitutes "low" for you may be different than what is considered low for someone else. So make sure the Doctor you are seeking a consult with is experienced and educated in truly understanding how to diagnose men who suffer from low testosterone. To find a list of some of the best TRT physicians available, visit this website: http://TRTDoctors.com

SYMPTOMS OF LOW TESTOSTERONE

THE most important consideration for whether a man should be on TRT is if they are experiencing "the symptoms" of low or below normal levels of testosterone.

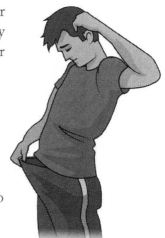

These can be any of the following:

1. Mental fog or loss of focus
2. Indecisiveness or hesitancy
3. Lack of energy
4. Decreased work performance
5. Decrease in sex drive or ability to reach orgasm
6. Decrease in strength or endurance
7. Decreased "enjoyment of life"
8. Noticeable change in behavior

If you have experienced any 4 of the following symptoms, you should strongly consider further testing and potentially TRT. I believe any critically-thinking man looking to optimize their health and well-being should be using TRT once their blood levels fall into the 'low normal' range. If your levels are below 'low', I see no other recourse but to seek out testosterone replacement therapy.

There are two commonly used questionnaires which are sometimes used as a diagnostic in men with symptoms of low testosterone: ADAM and AMS (They are never used in isolation due to their low specificity.)

ADAM (ANDROGEN DEFICIENCY IN AGING MALES)

This survey is a simple 10 questions survey[52] in yes or no format (the questionnaire is positive if there are yes answers to questions 1, 7 plus 3 other questions).

ANSWER YES OR NO TO EACH OF THE FOLLOWING QUESTIONS:

1. Do you have a decrease in libido (sex drive)?
2. Do you have a lack of energy?
3. Do you have a decrease in strength and/or endurance?
4. Have you lost height?
5. Have you noticed a decreased "enjoyment of life?"
6. Are you sad and/or grumpy?
7. Are your erections less strong?
8. Have you noticed a recent deterioration in your ability to play sports?
9. Are you falling asleep after dinner?
10. Has there been a recent deterioration in your work performance?

AMS (AGING MALES SYMPTOMS)

This survey[53] is much more detailed and divided into 3 quadrants-physical, psychological and sexual symptoms. It has 17 questions.

You can download it here:

www.aging-males-symptoms-scale.info/documents/question.pdf

Both of these questionnaires can be useful but they are only an adjunct to a proper *clinical diagnosis by an experienced TRT prescribing physician*.

---

52   http://www.prostatehealthnaturally.com/downloads/ADAM_Questionnaire.pdf

53   http://www.aging-males-symptoms-scale.info/documents/question.pdf

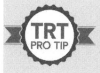

It sure would make a lot of sense for somebody in the clinician community to develop a questionnaire designed to monitor the success and or failure of ongoing testosterone replacement therapy.

Know Your Testosterone Levels, Understand Your Test Results

The most important objective consideration for TRT is if your measurement of "free" and "total serum" testosterone levels are low or out of range. Optimally, a man should exhibit testosterone levels at least at the highest end of the normal range (depending on the total testosterone measuring scale). The problem is what defines the 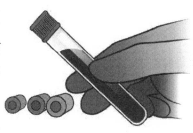 'normal range'? There is an infinite hormonal diversity across the male population and there is no real way to compress all men into a rigid 'standard patient' normal range model.

The following chart shows the variance ranges between the primary blood lab measurement companies.

Laboratory	Normal Range of Total Testosterone
LabCorp	348–1197 ng/dL
Quest Diagnostics	250–1100 ng/dL
Bio Reference Laboratories	300–1000 ng/dL

The biggest issue with these measurement companies is the variance of their assays between total and free testosterone levels in healthy young men.[54] While variation between laboratories for the same testosterone assay (analytical method) is negligible, the reference ranges for testosterone levels [as well as luteinizing hormone (**LH**) and follicle-

---

54   Bhasin, S., et al., The impact of assay quality and reference ranges on clinical decision making in the diagnosis of androgen disorders. Steroids, 2008. 73(13): p. 1311-7

stimulating hormone (**FSH**)] differ widely and significantly between assays.[55]

This means a critically thinking TRT-prescribing physician can't ultimately rely on blood levels provided by varying lab assays as an indicator of whether somebody qualifies for TRT or not. Clearly the flaws of laboratory analysis—either due to variation of hormonal production or the inaccuracy inherent to the testing methods—renders evaluation of a man's hormonal state, at times, more guesswork than science. Do you see the conundrum this presents for TRT prescribing physicians? The assumption there is a specific testosterone level threshold below which the symptoms appear, and the threshold is the same for everybody, is not an acceptable standard. There is far too much variance.

 Physicians should always treat the clinical presenting symptoms first. If you have blood levels in the normal to high range (usually above 500ng/dl), **YOU SHOULD NOT BE PUT ON TESTOSTERONE**. There are *always exceptions to the rule* but under normal circumstances a patient must possess not only low to low normal blood testosterone levels but 4-5 of the accepted low T symptoms before obtaining a prescription for TRT. Remember: This book is written in the context of HEALTH and LONGEVITY only. This is not a book about the prescribing or use of anabolic steroids or synthetics for performance enhancement. The Long Term Goal of TRT should be about improving quality of life.

---

55   Sikaris, K., et al., Reproductive hormone reference intervals for healthy fertile young men: evaluation of automated platform assays. J Clin Endocrinol Metab, 2005. 90(11): p. 5928-36.

HOW TO GET TESTED FOR LOW TESTOSTERONE

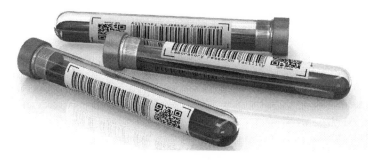

When working with a knowledgeable and experienced TRT physician, have him order your blood test. Realize the process may be slower and potentially more expensive (than from an online private lab measurement company) depending on whether you have a medical benefits plan. Just make sure to inform and engage your doctor about your long term goal of using TRT productively. Some doctors are more flexible in their criteria for justifying blood tests and will work with you to ensure everything is evaluated closely. I define and discuss the important lab assays (blood tests) needed in finer detail in Chapter 10.

Any doctor who provides unnecessary resistance to getting a blood test (let alone discussing TRT) is probably going to be troublesome and unhelpful to the process. If he or she is unwilling to intelligently discuss your request or rejects it out of hand, it is your right to seek the counsel of another doctor. When this happens (and it happens far too often) it usually indicates your doctor doesn't understand the importance of optimal testosterone levels and vitality. You now know conclusively symptoms can often trump blood values when dealing with low testosterone. It is imperative the doctor you work with is able to intelligently discuss your individual condition (respective of your blood panels and symptoms) and can formulate a sound and safe clinical diagnosis moving forward.

One simple and inexpensive preliminary way (before having your doctor order comprehensive labs) to measure your serum testosterone levels is to order a TRT blood test online. *It's easy, fast, convenient* and as simple as ordering a book from Amazon.com. You just go to the website, add the blood test to your cart, and checkout/pay.

After placing the order, you then go to the closest participating blood testing lab in your area (as referred to by the website) at a time that works with your schedule and get your blood drawn. The lab visit should take less than 10 minutes You'll receive your results typically within a few days via email. Just visit the website below to get all the details: http://TRTRev.com/blood-tests

It is a good idea before embarking down the long term path of TRT under the guidance of your physician to know your current blood Testosterone levels before getting started. Your TRT-prescribing doctor *should be able* to use these private lab results in making a diagnosis of whether or not you qualify for TRT. However if they will not accept them (and the test does reveal suboptimal blood testosterone levels) they are still an excellent discussion point in your initial consultation and conversation.

For men in their 20's and 30's fortunate enough to be undergoing TRT, I recommend you get your blood drawn at least once a year. For those of you in your 40's and up, twice a year is best. An Anti-Aging Panel is highly recommended for anybody 35 and up. You can get one here: http://TRTRev. com/anti-aging-panel

If you are not already doing so, you should begin regularly getting your blood work done so you can compile and reference all of your blood panel data for life. Having a detailed timeline from your very first/initial blood testosterone panel will provide excellent comparison points as your values and biomarkers change over time. And they will change without doubt. It is part of the process we call aging.

Obviously your physician will be documenting this but I also recommend you keeping copies of your blood panels yourself so you can become intimately aware of the changes you experience. Do your homework and know your body. I will be discussing the type of blood panels a progressive TRT-prescribing physician should be ordering along with the importance of monitoring them in Chapter 10.

TESTOSTERONE REPLACEMENT THERAPY NON-INJECTABLE OPTIONS

CHAPTER 6

There are a number of approved strategies for TRT. They differ and vary almost as much as the physicians administering them. Based on nearly 15 years of experimentation with every different type of TRT delivery system (while under the clinical care of doctors and also engaging and consulting with hundreds of men) I can transparently say not all of them are equal in their efficacy.

It is important to discuss the current and most accepted delivery systems so the reader can make an informed decision when comparing it to my preferred and recommended option.

There are many TRT-prescribing physicians who will disagree with this author's recommendation. It is important for the reader to understand this book is written as a guide for men who desire to optimally raise their testosterone to the higher end of the accepted range. My optimal protocol *doesn't ever* raise T levels to supraphysiologic levels often seen with anabolic steroid abusers. Many TRT prescribing clinicians are interested in restoring aging men to "normal" or "middle range" testosterone levels. Many of these folks are the primary prescribers of non injectable TRT. There is nothing wrong with such a strategy. In my opinion, my protocol does the best job of maximizing blood test levels (within accepted ranges) while improving health and minimizing side effects regardless of age. Maximizing blood test levels (while staying within accepted ranges) will provide the ultimate experience men are looking for when undergoing TRT.

The following chart outlines the current and accepted forms of TRT.

Testosterone Replacement Therapies Approved for Use in the USA					
Delivery System (Drug)	Route of Delivery	Standard Dosage for Androgen Deficiency	Advantages	Disadvantages	Estimated Monthly Cost
Testosterone Esters Testosterone enanthate Testosterone cypionate	Intermuscular	100 mg every week or 200 mg every 2 weeks	Inexpensive; administered every 2 weeks	Roller-coaster pharmacokinetics; requires injection	$65-95
Testosterone Pellets	Subcutaneous	Two to six 75-mg pellets every 3-6 months	Convenient 6-month biological duration	Expensive; requires small incision; high rate of extrusion; available only through manufacturer	$150
Buccal Testosterone	Buccal	30 mg BID (twice a day)	Testosterone levels within physiologic range	Expensive; twice-daily dosing; possible oral irritation	$250
Testosterone Patch	Nonscrotal topical	5 mg/day	Mimics circadian rhythm	Expensive; daily administration; skin irritation	$250
Testosterone Gel	Topical	5 g/day	Testosterone levels within physiologic range	Expensive; daily administration; possible transference to intimate contacts	$300

TRANSDERMAL CREAMS AND GELS (ANDROGEL)

Androgel is the #1 most prescribed TRT protocol in the world.[56] There are millions of men around the world using it. Many doctors believe in its therapeutic value in raising low testosterone. The gels come in either 1, 2, 5 and 10% concentrations and when applied in the morning produce 'physiologic serum levels.' In my opinion it's sub-optimal for a number of reasons. 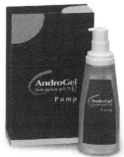 Primarily because it's difficult to control the delivery of the dosage often times leading to inadequate serum testosterone levels. In my opinion, absorption through the skin is inefficient due to food consumption, sweat glands, etc. Often times this inconsistent absorption rate produces an increase in DHT levels and potentially estrogenic side effects like puffy nipples, water retention and a sullen-moody temperament. It is also high risk when coming into contact with women or children.

In my experience it is a nuisance having to regularly apply creams or gels plus patients have to avoid swimming, bathing, showering and/or excess sweating for hours after application. Why would you want to constantly crimp your lifestyle to apply this to various regions of your body? Many men choose this method of TRT because it is the 'path of least resistance' both from a pain standpoint (injections) and because many doctors dispense this form cavalierly. I also have found it difficult to maintain stable blood values due to poor absorption rates. In my opinion, 1-2% creams/gels will never raise your testosterone levels to an optimal range that can be achieved with injectable formats.

---

56   Yu Z, Gupta SK, Hwang SS, et al. Testosterone pharmacokinetics after application of an investigational transdermal system in hypogonadal men. J Clin Pharmacol. 1997;37:1139–1145. [PubMed][Ref list]

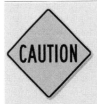

Dr. John Crisler, author of the excellent book *Testosterone Replacement Therapy-Recipe for Success*[57], believes transdermal delivery systems are superior to injectable formats. His belief is based on years of clinical experience with hundreds of patients. His theory is that transdermal delivery systems produce a serum androgen profile which varies greatly during the day-essentially mimicking the endogenous T production of a young healthy male. Better stated, entropy (randomness) in hormone levels best replicates the feelings of youth. Because they also elevate DHT, the transdermals are better at addressing sexual dysfunction[58].

TESTOSTERONE PELLETS

Pellets the size of 3 mm by 9 mm containing testosterone are surgically implanted under the skin (usually near the hip) and then slowly release testosterone over the course of 3-6 months.[59] Pellets are believed to have the longest duration of action of all forms of TRT on the 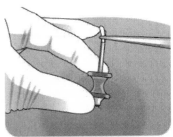 market today. Use of this form of therapy is suboptimal. First of all, there is a risk of infection and or hemorrhage at the point of insertion whenever anyone is exposed to surgery. It is also difficult to control the concentration of the dosage upon inserting the first pellets. If your blood levels indicate you need more or less of your dosage your physician will have to again perform invasive surgery to titrate therapy. Having to routinely have outpatient procedures to add or extract pellets is a nuisance. My recommendation is to consider a different form of TRT.

BIO-IDENTICAL TESTOSTERONE

57   http://www.trtrev.com/testosterone-recipe

58   Testosterone Replacement Therapy-A Recipe for Success-Dr. John Crisler pg.33 Milestones Publishing (March 13, 2015)

59   Kelleher S, Conway AJ, Handelsman DJ. Influence of implantation site and track geometry on the extrusion rate and pharmacology of testosterone implants. Clin Endocrinol.2001;55:531–536. [PubMed]

The term 'bio-identical' is often misconstrued. Even by physicians. It is often claimed bio-identical testosterone is "better" or more "natural" than pharmaceutical-grade testosterone. Case in point, "Bio-identical preparations are better because they're synthesized to be exactly like human testosterone circulating in the blood." UNTRUE. Pharmaceutical grade injectable testosterone IS bio-identical. It is an "esterified" form of testosterone. In other words, testosterone is attached to a carrier molecule (the ester) which is enzymatically cleaved (broken off), leaving testosterone, the "identical" molecule that your gonads produce.

The fact that a testosterone preparation (testosterone cypionate, for example) is pharmaceutical grade, DOES NOT equate to it being a potentially dangerous "synthetic," the all-too-often abused substance of bodybuilders. "Synthetics" are NON-bio-identical testosterone-like substances, synthesized in the lab (or potentially in someone's garage) which promote anabolism. Foreign to the body (unlike bio-identicals), synthetics put the user at risk for a whole host of dangerous side effects (liver dysfunction and cancer, for example). I do not advocate the usage of synthetics. The risks simply outweigh the benefits. This is about health after all, right? This is NOT about bodybuilding.

BUCCAL PREPARATIONS

This method is applying a tablet of oral testosterone medication twice daily to your gums so it absorbs into your bloodstream. Known as a "cyclodextrin-complexed tes-tosterone sublingual formulation" or a tro-che, this form of TRT is absorbed rapidly 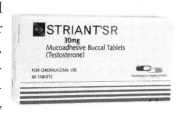 into circulation while the testosterone is released from the cyclodextrin shell.[60] Not only is this an inefficient method of getting testosterone into your system, but the potential side effects of dislodged tablets, bleeding gums, mouth sores, toothaches and headaches make it ill advised. Plus

---

60   Salehian B, Wang C, Alexander G, et al. Pharmacokinetics, bioefficacy, and safety of sublingual testosterone cyclodextrin in hypogonadal men: comparison to testosterone enanthate – a clinical research center study. J Clin Endocrinol Metab. 1995;80:3567–3575. [PubMed]

the ability to transfer the substance to your partner via kissing is way too risky. And what about the issue of ingested foods and liquids combining with the buccal testosterone preparation? Again, my recommendation is to choose a better form of TRT.

PATCHES

Transdermal testosterone is also available as a scrotal skin patch. Scrotal patches produce high levels of dihydrotestosterone (DHT) due to high 5-alpha-reductase enzyme activity of scrotal skin.[61] This is a BIG NO NO as high levels of DHT are to be avoided due to their ability to produce unwanted side effects like acne, hair loss and potential prostate issues in select individuals.

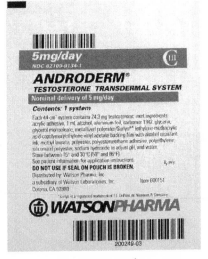

This form of TRT can also cause skin irritation at place of adhesion. What man wants to be caught in an intimate situation with a woman while wearing a scrotal patch? Really? I think you should pass on this delivery system.

All of these TRT options work, but in my opinion are far from optimal. Their benefits do not outweigh their potential side effects. This book is written for men who want to excel in all phases of life via optimal testosterone levels. Why would men looking to become more empowered and physically optimal want TRT preparations so mild they only raise testosterone levels to the 'normal range'? In addition their poor absorption and administration rates are potentially irritating, painful and a nuisance. They often convert to DHT which leads to unwanted side effects. No thanks.

---

61   Kim MK, Zhao H, Lee CH, Kim DD. Formulation of a reservoir-type testosterone transdermal delivery system. Int J Pharm. 2001;219(1–2):51–59. [PubMed]

TRT Via Intramuscular Injection and My Optimal TRT Protocol

Chapter 7

As I've intimated previously, any legitimate TRT physician should explore all options to find the stressor or cause of low testosterone before initiating actual testosterone replacement therapy (especially with men under the age of 30 looking to remain fertile).

Understanding this, the three recommended vital life markers 'that should be" met before beginning TRT:

1. **Age 30 or older** (if younger, proceed with caution, do your homework and make sure you're financially able). You must also find and work with a progressive TRT-prescribing physician willing to work with you should your presenting symptoms and blood levels warrant a low T diagnosis).

2. **Testosterone levels lower than 500 on a verifiable blood test** (it really depends on your SYMPTOMS if at the higher end of this "low normal" range. Also remember different blood test companies provide varying range lab assay values that differ widely and significantly[62]) Physicians should NEVER chase lab numbers and clearly evaluate symptoms first and foremost.

3. **Experiencing 4 or more of the symptoms of what is recognized as low testosterone.**

Ultimately your physician is evaluating your **clinical symptoms** as his final determinant for diagnosis. Symptoms are the MOST

---

62   Bhasin, S., et al., The impact of assay quality and reference ranges on clinical decision making in the diagnosis of androgen disorders. Steroids, 2008. 73(13): p. 1311-7

IMPORTANT determinant of whether a man should begin a TRT regimen.

If these all apply to you, it is reasonable to consider you a candidate for TRT.

INTRAMUSCULAR INJECTION (IM)

As previously discussed, there are many ways to increase testosterone via various TRT protocols. Although a topic often debated inside anti-aging, endocrinology and TRT-prescribing circles, I believe (based on nearly 15 years of experience with every TRT delivery system) the single most effective form of TRT to optimize testosterone blood values is via injection. There is recent scientific evidence also supporting my opinion[63].

There are four main types of injectable testosterone formulations found on the market today.

TESTOSTERONE CYPIONATE AND TESTOSTERONE ENANTHATE

The majority of TRT-prescribing physicians prescribe *80–200 mg doses of injectable testosterone cypionate and testosterone enanthate every 7–21 days.* The mg dosage amounts vary depending on the doctor and their individual methodologies. This is an observed protocol of many TRT-prescribing clinicians for the following reasons:

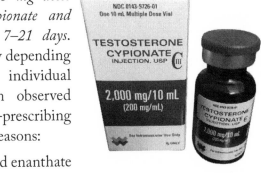

- Because cypionate and enanthate enjoy longer half-lives, they allow the user to minimize their injection frequency.
- Many men have needle phobia and don't want to administer frequent injections. Nor do doctors want their staff/nurses to prepare multiple monthly injections for their clients and then send them in the mail (when working with clients virtually).

63   Injection of Testosterone May be Safer and More Effective than Transdermal Administration for Combating Loss of Muscle and Bone in Older men-Stephen E. Borst and Joshua F. Yarrow-Am J Physiol Endocrinol Metab (April 21, 2015)

Imagine the liability potentially faced with some inexperienced patient who can't inject himself.

- It is also much more convenient for a man to visit his doctor's office once a week for his weekly or every-other-weekly injection than it is for him to come daily or inject himself daily (despite many diabetics who are accustomed to injecting themselves on a daily basis with insulin).
- Enanthate and cypionate are mass-produced by compounding pharmacies and their wholesale cost is WAY CHEAPER.

Testosterone cypionate and enanthate are virtually identical in release patterns and there is little difference between the two chemically. The ester found in both has an active half-life between 5 (enanthate) and 6 (cypionate) days but blood levels fall sharply 4 days after administration.[64]

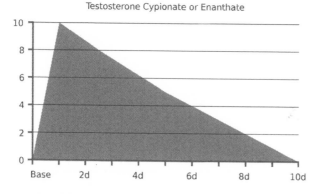

Testosterone Cypionate or Enanthate

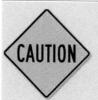

Patients are often prescribed what I believe to be inadequate 80-100 mg doses of cypionate or enanthate injected once every 14-21 days. This creates wide swings in serum androgen levels. As already mentioned above, the result is too many peaks and valleys of both testosterone and estrogen causing an emotional up and down feeling due to the lack of balance between the two hormones. Patients are then prescribed an *aromatization inhibitor* (AI) like Arimidex (Anastrozole) as a result to fix the

64   Dobs AS, Meikle AW, Arver S, Sanders SW, Caramelli KE, Mazer NA. Pharmacokinetics, efficacy, and safety of a permeation enhanced testosterone transdermal system in comparison with bi-weekly injections of testosterone enanthate for the treatment of hypogonadal men. J Clin Endocrinol Metab. 1999;84:3469–3478. [PubMed]

problem of increased estrogen inadvertently created from the dosing schedule. It is very rare (except in specific cases of high body fat individuals or older men) that a patient should be started out on an aromatase inhibitor (AI). The need for estrogen control must be proven first. This is why follow up labs are crucial to understand what is really going on in that individuals endocrine system as a response to using supplemental T.

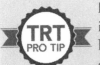 It is the author's opinion it is imperative when undergoing TRT one avoids the peaks and valleys often caused by longer acting (half-life) testosterone esters dosed too infrequently. This produces what many prescribing physicians observe as a roller coaster effect of rapid fluctuations in plasma estrogen (E) and testosterone (T).[65] How can the mass prescribing of cypionate/enanthate be beneficial under this "normal TRT protocol" of one shot every 14–21 Days? Clearly it is not.

The most progressive TRT prescribing physicians are doing a much better job of administering cypionate and enanthate by utilizing 1-2x a week injection protocols and also providing the correct dosage necessary (80-200mgs every 7-10 days depending on patient response) to minimize peaks and valleys. Dr. John Crisler adamantly recommends (and I agree) T injections be administered at a maximum frequency of 7 days. I would also point out it is IMPERATIVE when first beginning a TRT protocol, no other medications which manipulate hormone levels (AI's) be dosed (except for hCG potentially) to find out how the testosterone dose affects that person's endocrine system by itself. Once follow up labs are received, it may be practical to start a patient on an AI if aromatase inhibition is warranted. There are exceptions to this rule further discussed in Chapter 9.

---

65   Behre HM, et al. Pharmacology of testosterone preparations. In: Nieschlag E, Behre HM, editors. Testosterone, action, deficiency, substitution. Cambridge University Press; 2004. pp. 405–44.

Testosterone Undecanoate

This injectable testosterone preparation is better known as Nebido and is used in Europe and Scandinavian countries. Recently, Aveed of Endo Pharmaceuticals[66] has become available in the US. Theoretically, it is a perfect formulation because it has a very long half-life and is injected only once every 10 to 14 weeks.[67] In practice, many men who have used it claim to suffer from the normal 'valleys' expected from a longer acting testosterone ester losing its effectiveness toward weeks 7–10. It

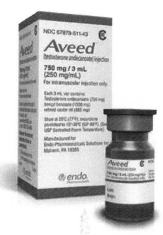

has also anecdotally been found to rarely raise testosterone levels above the midrange of 'normal' (when measured between 4-8 weeks into therapy). What is most concerning is the idea of having higher estrogen with very little exogenous testosterone left from the original injection while waiting for the next injection to come. Aveed as of recent report, is now allowing clinicians to titrate therapy by decreasing the duration between injections. I believe this form of TRT has a promising future but does not rival my optimal and recommended protocol currently.

A newer oral capsule form of Testosterone Undecanoate, **Rextoro** has recently applied for FDA approval but was rejected. In theory it too offers great promise as it is absorbed via the lymphatic system bypassing the liver.

It should also be noted Aveed's website offers a very stern warning of the risk of "serious pulmonary microembolism (POME) reactions and anaphylaxis" upon injection. This is due to the chemical particulates in the injectable formulation (to extend its half-life) being potentially harmful to some users.

---

66   http://www.aveedusa.com/

67   Von Eckardstein, Nieschlag E. Treatment of male hypogonadism with testosterone undecanoate injected at extended intervals of 12 weeks: a phase II study. J Androl.2002;23(3):419–425. [PubMed]

TESTOSTERONE PROPIONATE

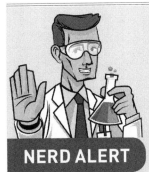 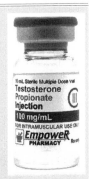

Testosterone propionate is a fast-acting, short half-life (2.25 days) testosterone ester. The testosterone ester determines how long it takes your body to dispose of the hormone in question and propionate is one of the shortest esters available with a testosterone base. There are

NERD ALERT

enzymes in the body called 'esterases' which are responsible for removing the ester from testosterone. Once the ester is removed, all that is left is just the testosterone molecule itself. The longer the ester, the longer testosterone is active in the body and the less overall testosterone dosage is absorbed.

Because of testosterone propionate's short half-life, peak blood levels can be modulated via injection frequency. When dosed daily or every-other-day (EOD) propionate can mimic the testosterone your body naturally produces. Its half-life is shorter than the longer-acting esters of cypionate and enanthate. In fact, after a single injection of 50 mg, the maximum concentration is reached after approximately 14 hours.[68]

The chart below shows how much testosterone is absorbed and used for each 100 mg injected. Depending on the weight of the ester, the injectable formulations deliver different net bioavailable mg amounts. For example, if you inject 100 mg of testosterone undecanoate, only 63 mg of it will be available for use by the body.

100 mg of injectable as:	Approximate Free Equivalent (how much actually gets used by the body from a 100 mg dosage):
Testosterone Propionate	83 mg
Testosterone Enanthate	72 mg
Testosterone Cypionate	70 mg
Testosterone Undecanoate	63 mg

68   Behre HM, et al. Pharmacology of testosterone preparations. In: Nieschlag E, Behre HM, editors. Testosterone, action, deficiency, substitution. Cambridge University Press; 2004. pp. 405–44

As you can see testosterone propionate is the most effective formulation (from a peak concentration standpoint on a mg per mg basis) found on the market today.

It has recently come to my attention the DEA may frown upon the dispensing of testosterone propionate instead of testosterone cypionate or enanthate by physicians. The reason given: "it is used more often for performance optimization like GH (growth hormone) and is a red flag". I can absolutely verify there are numerous physicians prescribing testosterone propionate in their practices without issue. This may warrant further monitoring for any patient or doctor using testosterone propionate.

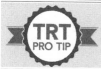 **30-50 mgs of Testosterone Propionate injected every other day (EOD) is an excellent option and my recommended protocol for long term TRT administration.**

In lieu of the DEA's recent stance on the usage of Testosterone Propionate and the possibility of your TRT prescribing physician being unable to script it, the preferred alternative would be a *Cypionate/ Enanthate dosage protocol of 50-100 mgs every 3rd day*. For those patients who are extremely needle phobic, you can do one intramuscular injection of 100-200 mgs every 7th day (once per week) instead.

It is important to maintain 7 days as the maximum time between shots (100-200 mgs dosage) and hence why two shots (50-100 mgs per dosage) every seven days is optimal. The "right dosage" is an individual thing and it will require you and your doctor testing levels of T and E to establish and maintain balance. Balance should be defined as feeling great with minimal to no side effects.

As is continually stated in this book, if you live in a country or state where it is illegal to administer testosterone without a doctor's prescription, then choosing the route of self-administration without a legitimate prescription is breaking the law. I do not assume any liability for the information presented. I urge all of my readers to educate themselves on the laws of their respective country or state.

THE FDA IS NOT THE ENEMY

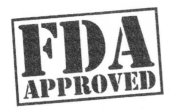

The United States FDA (Food and Drug Administration) is a very difficult agency to predict behaviorally. In 2014 it appeared they were effectually attempting to "narrow the official approval guidelines for testosterone replacement therapy" when their expert panels[69] urged them to limit the indication for prescribing TRT "to men whose low testosterone stems from an acute medical problem such as damaged testicles or thyroid disease."

But then a recent 2014 ruling by the very same FDA[70] rebutted anti-HRT studies claiming HRT increases the risk of cardiovascular disease. They were actually responding to a petition filed by two physicians, Drs. Wolfe and Carome, who were asking for the FDA to force a black box warning on testosterone products that would state increased CVD (cardiovascular disease) risks[71]. Strangely enough, on March 3, 2015 the FDA contradicted their previous rebuttal[72] when they ruled testosterone products will require those very same labels "to clarify that the prescription hormone is meant for use by men whose low testosterone levels are caused by certain medical conditions," such as

---

69 http://www.hcplive.com/articles/Will-the-FDA-Tighten-the-Use-of-Testosterone-Replacement-Therapy

70 http://www.peaktestosterone.com/Testosterone_FDA.aspx

71 http://www.peaktestosterone.com/FDA_Denial_Petition_July%2016_2014.pdf

72 http://www.latimes.com/science/sciencenow/la-sci-sn-testosterone-heart-stroke-risk-20150303-story.html

"genetic disorders and conditions affecting the testicles, pituitary gland and brain."

In truth, the data upon which the FDA based its ruling is relevant to a select group of individuals: men over 65 years of age with pre-existing heart conditions. Obviously, it cannot be applied to the general population of men supplementing with testosterone.

Bottom line: It is not only appropriate but safe to place warnings on medications to alert those who may be at risk for side effects. Do ALL MALES fall into this high-risk category? Are the 2 million plus Americans currently on testosterone therapy destined to develop atherosclerotic heart disease? Of course not! In fact, there are over 50 RECENT STUDIES[73] demonstrating testosterone's profound cardioprotective effects. Links to some of this data are provided and thoroughly discussed in Chapter 10.

I wish I could say this is surprising but TRT appears to remain an FDA lightning rod of scrutiny maintaining the gray area of male hormone replacement therapy (HRT). It should make all men more steadfast in seeking the care and guidance of a highly qualified TRT prescribing physician. A physician not only able to counsel them intelligently regarding their care, but capable of advising them within the confines of the current and often changing laws.

CHOOSING THE RIGHT TRT-PRESCRIBING PHYSICIAN

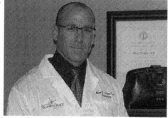

Often times the primary objective of our medical industry is to treat disease via medicating symptoms. The intentions of the men reading this book should be for fine tuning and optimizing TRT for maximum performance in all levels of their lives. These same men should be looking for an experienced TRT doctor knowledgeable in fine-tuning their endocrine system to run as efficiently as possible, forever.

As a result of their lack of experience and knowledge in this newer and specific realm of TRT, many doctors struggle to prescribe TRT for optimal health. Be wary of taking advice from a doctor who is not

---

73   http://www.ncbi.nlm.nih.gov/pmc/?term=Testosterone+is+Cardio+Protective

also using TRT and exhibiting the same benefits you are seeking. You'd ideally want to work with a doctor who practices what he preaches. Think twice about listening to the advice of a doctor who is obese, out of shape, or looks like he has not exercised a day in his life. If he is giving advice on how to take testosterone to improve your life, then he should be living proof of the success of its use. Would you take financial advice on how/where to invest your money from a college graduate who has a bachelor degree in finance? Or from an entrepreneur/investor who has a multi-million dollar investment portfolio?

It is also important to understand the potential costs of long-term TRT before beginning. The fees TRT physicians charge will vary.

On the more expensive side, an anti-aging clinic can charge as much as a $250-1,250 initial consultation fee along with a monthly membership fee ($100-500) to allow their patients to obtain a prescription for testosterone, other anti-aging meds and concierge access to the physician.

Alternatively, others can charge a fee to speak with a doctor or nurse. Medications are prescribed so that you can be reimbursed through your medical benefit plan (when allowed). In some instances, medical treatments are offered conveniently through a telemedicine platform allowing the patient to consult with expert TRT physicians virtually via webcam, phone, and email so that you don't have to travel far to get affordable treatment. Visit the website below for more details:

http://TRTRev.com/defy

To view a comprehensive list of recommended anti-aging and TRT practitioners, visit www.TRTDoctors.com

As I will continue to say throughout this book, do your research when it comes to choosing this course of action.

CHAPTER 7 READER QUESTIONS

What is the optimal form of TRT for a newbie starting out?

Whatever a knowledgeable TRT prescribing physician believes is in your best interest based on your blood test results and their clinical diagnosis from your presenting symptoms. Optimally, using Testosterone Cypionate or Enanthate at between 80-200 mgs per week should be more than enough for any adult male to elevate their T levels to the highest end of the range with minimal side effects. It is my opinion as a TRT user becomes more experienced they can experiment with increased frequency of injections and possibly using testosterone propionate when able to be scripted without issue.

My doctor recommends Nebido and argues it is far superior to all other Esters. He is an author of a standard endocrinology textbook and head of the WHO Center for andrology at the university hospital of Muenster. What do you think about Nebido or Aveed?

First of all I'm very familiar with your Professor Eberhard Nieschlag and his comprehensive 2012 textbook **Testosterone: Action, Deficiency, Substitution**[74]. There are actually citations from his research in this book.

Nebido and Aveed are actually testosterone undecanoate. An old-school version of testosterone just re-engineered as an injectable format today. It used to be available under the trade name 'Andriol' and it was in capsule form. It's actually a very weak and mild form of testosterone (actually quite expensive too) but there are no observed side effects from its use on the HPTA/HPGA. Supposedly it doesn't disturb follicle-stimulating hormone (FSH) or luteinizing hormone (LH) either. Nebido has been used in parts of Europe for more than a decade. As I already wrote in Chapter 6, the jury is still out even though it theoretically shows promise. The biggest issue I have is the injection volume at initial dosing being either 750 mgs or 1,000 mgs. That is a lot of injection volume. With that much injection volume there is a risk of pain at the injection point or even injecting into a blood vessel. Aveed is tough to come by in the USA because in order to have it prescribed your physician must be registered and certified by Endo Pharmaceuticals and their REMS (Risk Evaluation and Mitigation Strategy). REMS is a very strict form of post marketing surveillance designed to note and record any adverse effects associated with Aveed.

On a long enough time horizon (months), is there really any difference between test cyp and test prop if you inject both at least 3x/week (given the same amount of test equivalents)?

As far as efficacy, mg-for-mg, it probably won't matter as much. I'd bet that if you did blood work for 7 days in a row, you'd have elevated testosterone levels each day you were on prop. And you'd have days without elevated doses when on cyp. So there may or may not be a marginal benefit to using prop since you'd be at higher levels every day. Those days of having higher levels should add up.

Would testosterone cypionate (E3D) be more optimal (and convenient) than propionate (EOD) since the peaks and valleys are closer together?

This is essentially my recommended protocol. But to answer your specific question, testosterone is essentially testosterone. There is no reason to concern yourself with half-lives in the way you're thinking. What you want to minimize are side effects. Cypionate might make you hold more water. It's not as fast-acting (in the response you 'FEEL') and it also won't clear your system as fast as propionate will. Plus propionate (due to it's short half life) mimics your body's natural production much more closely than cypionate/enanthate.

I'm 54 and have been doing Testosterone Enanthate 250 1/2 cc twice weekly for about 18 months, and have no side effects at all. Blood work came back great. I have never been in better shape. Lost like 20 lbs of fat and leaned out really nice. Two questions—can I maintain this dose forever? Also if I were to come off should I consider a PTC Cycle and if so what would you recommend?

There is no reason to come off ever! And at 54 why would you? You have very little natural production at this stage of your life and I assume you aren't wanting kids. There is much more info on why cycling Testosterone is ineffective in Chapter 10.

Consider utilizing medications that keep your HPTA/HPGA working like *hCG/hMG* (discussed in detail in Chapter 10) These medications may be necessary should you have any down regulation of your HPTA/HPGA. Again, I stress utilizing the services of a competent TRT prescribing physician to treat and hopefully prevent/control any issues or side effects.

I just had my blood work done yesterday at a local anti-aging clinic. My question is actually in regards to hCG. Recently I noticed on various boards, where guys have actually posted their labs showing on hCG and off, and one guy had as much as a 400 mg difference being on it as compared to off of it. Is this BS? Or does its impact vary from person to person?

Science is really primitive and deals with large populations when we all have different genes and our genes express themselves in different ways.

Here's what I mean. Answer this: does zinc raise testosterone? Normally, no it does not. But for some men, zinc does raise their testosterone levels. Placebo? No. It's genes. Even how some guys respond to testosterone is based on genotype. If you have a lot of androgen receptors in your traps, TRT will give you big traps. So does hCG raise testosterone? In a population-wide study? It may or may not. Will it raise yours? It might.

Someday everyone with money will have his genes mapped out. Then you'll be able to take medications aimed at targeting how your individual body works. Until then all you can do is rely on general guidelines and use your brain and try things out on yourself. Hence why I am so vigilant on getting regular blood work. Blood work. Try something. More blood work. Analyze.

Then you figure this stuff out and find out what works ideally for you. We all have unique biochemical individuality. *hCG* monotherapy (discussed in detail in Chapter 10) is used by physicians to elevate testosterone levels. There is research indicating it does work especially with younger men who don't want to disturb their endogenous (natural) testosterone production. Dr. John Crisler recommends *hCG* at 250-500 iu per shot on the last 2 days of a once a week injection week (known as

The Crisler Method)[75]. hCG can also be used daily at 100 iu's with great success due to its ability to produce randomness in the serum androgen profile at varying points in the day. You can learn more about Dr. John Crisler here: http://TRTRev.com/crisler

I'm 29. I have a very positive outlook on life. Always optimistic and looking forward to the next day. Sex drive is good, though at times a little indifferent, certainly not like it was 5–8 years ago. My body is in solid shape, training at the gym 3–5x/week and playing basketball 1–2x/week. I generally find myself sore the next day and slower out of bed after an intense workout or game. Blood pressure is low, and I eat clean. I'll admit that I was a bit disappointed by the numbers (testosterone is 409 and free testosterone is 83.8), but they probably jive with my overall demeanor. The numbers aren't surprising to me. Any thoughts about short term/long term prognosis?

I believe TRT is about treating symptoms, not numbers. Forget your number. How do you feel? If you feel great, you don't need to go on TRT. It's always a personal decision and hopefully one you make for valid reasons. Your numbers are low enough that you can reasonably investigate TRT. But again, it comes down to how you feel. Based on everything you've said above, I would investigate TRT further.

If I am injecting 1 ml per week and am coming up for a blood test, how long should I wait after doing the injection before going to the lab for the test?

You want to get your labs done when peak plasma values are attained. Is that 1 ml of testosterone cypionate? If so, peak values are generally attained 2 to 5 days after the injection. Take your dose on Monday and get blood work done on Thursday or Friday.

---

75   Testosterone Replacement Therapy-A Recipe for Success-Dr. John Crisler pg.71 Milestones Publishing (March 13, 2015)

I hear the term HRT (hormone replacement therapy) a lot. Is that for women? How is TRT different/same as HRT?

HRT as defined by Wikipedia:

"any form of hormone therapy wherein the patient, in the course of medical treatment, receives hormones, either to supplement a lack of naturally occurring hormones, or to substitute other hormones for naturally occurring hormones."

The term is definitely more visible in women's circles as hormone replacement for pre – and postmenopausal women. It involves the use of one or more medications designed to artificially boost hormone levels. The main types of hormones involved are estrogens, progesterone/progestins, and sometimes testosterone.

It is my opinion testosterone can be an effective woman's treatment for many of the same reasons it is so highly effective in men. As I stated in the preface of the book there is plenty of scientific evidence TRT for women[76] is highly effective and safe.[77] There are WAY too many proven myths surrounding women and TRT. I believe it warrants an entire book unto itself. Visit this website for more details:

http://TRTRev.com/women

How much of a hassle is it to go from being self medicated to being under a doctor's care?

This is an excellent question. It really depends on where you're being self medicated? Are you in the USA? How much does it cost you to procure T, ancillaries and to regularly get your blood work? It is crucially important to find a doctor who is willing to not only prescribe testosterone, but also monitor you properly.

There are some affluent patients that prefer to work with a professional the caliber of Dr. Brett Osborn: http://TRTRev.com/osborn. Then there are others that prefer a more affordable virtual telemedicine solution through Defy Medical: http://TRTRev.com/defy

---

76   Tuiten A, Von Honk J, Koppeschaar H, et al. Time course of effects of testosterone administration on sexual arousal in women. Arch Gen Psychiatry. 2000;57(2):149-153.

77   Davis SR. Cardiovascular and cancer safety of testosterone in women. Curr Opin Endocrinol Diabetes Obes. 2011;18(3):198-203.

If you have medical benefits, many of the anti-aging medications (Metformin, Armour Thyroid) and TRT ancillaries like (Arimidex, hCG, Nolvadex or Clomid) can be billed through insurance. Some of the meds will be more expensive than others and sometimes denied depending on your individual diagnosis (age) and the level of coverage you have.

As heavily discussed throughout this book, it is IMPERATIVE any man (or woman for that matter) do their homework and know thyself when it comes to supplementing with exogenous hormones. You MUST use a progressive and forward thinking physician who can counsel you through your attempts to find balance between T and E. No dosage nor reaction/response to said dosage is universal. It is like Dr. John Crisler states, 'dropping a pebble into an ocean.' The more you know about using TRT and how it may or may not affect your individual biochemistry, the higher your chances of long term success.

Furthermore, if you live in a country or state where it is illegal to administer testosterone without a doctor's prescription, then choosing the route of self-administration without a legitimate prescription is breaking the law.

THE INS AND OUTS OF PROPER INJECTION PROCEDURES

CHAPTER 8

Understanding my recommended protocol can involve one to multiple weekly injections, it is important we discuss and analyze the injection process. If working with an experienced and knowledgeable TRT physician, you will have the choice to self administer the injections (with their approval).

I don't know of many men choosing to make TRT a lifelong commitment (why would you not) not self administering their testosterone as well as *hCG*. In fact it is the most convenient option especially for those with busy lifestyles. Self injection just becomes a regular part of your day-to-day existence similar to brushing your teeth in the morning and night.

I want to emphasize there is no need to worry about injecting yourself. The 'pain' experienced is no worse than pinching the skin on the back of your hand. After receiving a couple of injections from your physician, physician's nurse (or even performing them yourself) you'll not even notice it. Some men have a 'needle phobia' upon their first injection. This is a perfectly acceptable psychological reaction. It vanishes once you realize there is minimal pain and less to worry about.

SYRINGE, NEEDLE GAUGE AND WITHDRAWING

There are many different sizes of syringes. To keep the math/conversion of your testosterone dosage simple, I recommend your physician providing a 3 ml syringe so it can be easily prepared to the correct mg/cc testosterone dosage. If at all possible, ask your physician to pre-load your TRT injections for you.

The barrel portion of the syringe will have units of measure from ½ – 3 ml (ticks marks) along the side. In terms of the actual size (diameter) of the needle, a 23-26 gauge 1' needle syringe is optimal. It is much easier to withdraw the testosterone solution with an 18 gauge 1½ withdrawing needle.

For men who have higher body fat percentages (over 20%), you are likely going to have to inject with a *25 gauge needle that is 1.5 inches long.* You'll have to penetrate beyond your visceral fat to make sure you inject into your muscle. This is another reason to focus on losing excess body fat to better optimize an injectable testosterone delivery system.

WHERE AND HOW TO INJECT SAFELY

With the syringe as your intramuscular injection (IM) tool, it is easy to inject testosterone into the following muscle areas: deltoids, gluteus, or upper/outside quadriceps. I recommend rotating your injection sites to minimize scar tissue formation. With essentially three different areas on each side of the body, you'll have up to 6 different places you can routinely inject. Visit this website for some great resources to understand proper injection procedures and technique: http://TRTRev.com/inject

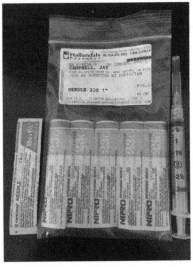

Just as there is no reason to fear intramuscular injections as causing pain, usage of the words 'minimizing scar tissue' isn't anything to worry about either. 23-26 gauge needles are minimally invasive upon injection. It is observed some TRT dispensing physicians will provide preloaded syringes for their patients. There is no reason not to ask your doctor to provide you a 1-month or even 10-week supply of preloaded T syringes (if your script is for 200 mgs for 10 cc's in Testosterone Cypionate or Enanthate).

TRT Via Subcutaneous Administration

Anecdotally, various men have reported great results (recently) following a TRT protocol of injecting subcutaneously. This is injecting into the fat tissue of the lower stomach or gluteal fat pad (buttocks) area with an insulin syringe (similarly to hCG). There is recent research indicating subcutaneous TRT produced therapeutic serum concentrations at doses generally lower than required for IM injections[78]. In other words (according to one study), less testosterone needs to be injected subcutaneously to achieve optimal T blood levels than intramuscular TRT. Both Dr. Eugene Shippen and Dr. John Crisler are using subcutaneous injection protocols with hundreds of patients. Dr. Crisler has found 40 mgs Testosterone Cypionate twice weekly to be as efficacious as 100 mg Cypionate intramuscularly (IM)[79]

Let's analyze this more closely. Isn't subcutaneously really intramuscular if the person has low body fat? It is easy to understand why some clinicians (and their patients) might favor the idea of 'less irritation and hole poking' from a small thin insulin needle injected into fat tissue. It is also apparent from our research, more frequent injections *might* equal less aromatization, lower blood levels of SHBG and better mimicking the body's natural production of testosterone. We could make a valid argument, if one felt injecting into their lower stomach quadrant was OK, it provides an additional injection spot to insert into their rotation of injection site areas.

---

78   Evaluation of the efficacy of subcutaneous administration of testosterone in female to male transexuals and hypogonadal males – – Olshan et al. 34 (3): MON-594 – – Endocrine Reviews

79   Testosterone Replacement Therapy-A Recipe for Success-Dr. John Crisler pg.99 Milestones Publishing (March 13, 2015)

It is my opinion injecting testosterone subcutaneously may or may not be as effective due to the potential aromatization of the testosterone in adipocytes (fat tissue). This is especially true for men who have excess body fat in their belly and love handle regions. Remember aromatase loves to 'hang out' in fat tissue[80]. Injecting testosterone into men with higher regional body fat deposition *might* be a recipe for estradiol (E2) conversion and the resulting negative side effects that come with it. Whatever your feeling of subcutaneous injections, it is a very cutting edge and apparently promising delivery system that merits close scrutiny and more observational study for current and future TRT users.

Once you're done injecting, throw the syringe away. Do NOT reuse syringes for hygienic purposes. Be smart about where you place your unused and used syringes. The most intelligent and hygienic way to dispose of your used insulin syringes is purchasing a Sharps Container Biohazard Needle Disposal[81]. Keep your syringes out of the reach of children for obvious reasons. Part of using TRT responsibly is simple common sense.

MINIMIZING SCAR TISSUE FORMATION WITH FOAM ROLLING AND MYOFASCIAL RELEASE

Using a foam roller[82] and/or a Beastie Ball[83] are essential home tools to break up scar tissue at injection sites. Just a couple times a week for about 2-5 minutes is enough. But as you work out and build larger muscle fibers, you'll definitely want to use

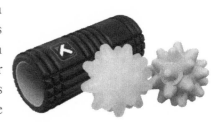

---

80   Intra-adipose sex steroid metabolism and body fat distribution in idiopathic human obesity. Clin Endocrinol (Oxf). 2007 Mar;66(3):440-6.

81   http://trtrev.com/sharps

82   http://trtrev.com/foam

83   http://trtrev.com/beastie

them more frequently to relieve muscle tightness and assist recovery so your muscles are flexible, healthy, and supple[84].

Whenever possible, supplement your at-home treatment with a deep tissue massage – **Active Release Technique** (ART) – by a professional massage therapist a couple times a month. Active Release Technique massage is an incredible way to improve full-body muscle elasticity and also to speed tissue recovery and healing. It is also a great adjunct to enhance strength and flexibility.[85]

Don't let the words scar tissue scare you. I'm talking about 'fascial adhesions'[86]. These are tiny micro-traumas that have built up from years of local injections into the muscle. They are rarely noticeable or even felt, but it's an excellent course of action to have an Active Release massage therapist (ART) break them up so they don't harden and solidify over time. Using foam rollers and the Beastie Ball will also help as a personal form of therapy.

84   http://fabfitover40.com/2014/06/25/key-to-remaining-fit-over-40/

85   DiGiovanna, Eileen; Schiowitz, Stanley; Dowling, Dennis J. (2005) [1991]. "Ch. 12: Myofascial (Soft Tissue) Techniques". An Osteopathic Approach to Diagnosis and Treatment (3rd ed.). Philadelphia: Lippincott Williams & Wilkins. pp. 80–2.

86   http://destroychronicpain.wordpress.com/fascial-adhesions-2/

CHAPTER 8 READER QUESTIONS

Will it be an issue going through airports and countries traveling with testosterone and syringes? Do I need to have a prescription with me?

You should have a copy of your prescription or at least have your medications indicated with the prescription labeling on the packaging and storage bag. It is unlikely to ever be an issue. For convenience purposes, pack your TRT equipment in your checked baggage using something like this diabetic organizer bag.

What if I develop a rash around my injection site?

It is possible to experience an allergic reaction from the chemical keeping the testosterone ester stable in injectable solution form (usually ethyl oleate or propylene glycol). Very rarely, an allergic reaction to an injection will lead to a localized skin infection. Often known as cellulitis, these are noticed as a burning sensation at the point of injection. Sometimes the skin turns red or fills with white blood cells. If you are experiencing these symptoms, it may be prudent to see your doctor. In the worst case scenario (and this is rarely seen or experienced), your doctor might have you do a round of antibiotics for several days to treat the cellulitis.

About a day after injection, I'm getting some soreness/bruising at the place where I injected. Is that normal? I just recently started TRT.

As a newbie to TRT, when first receiving intramuscular injections, you may experience minor soreness at the point of injection several hours later, almost like the soreness you'd feel if someone punched you in the arm. Most of the time you will feel nothing, but either way it's nothing to worry about and you'll just get used to it, eventually feeling no sensitivity at all.

I've heard from other TRT Patients they use a 28-31 gauge 5/16 Insulin Syringe to inject their testosterone intramuscularly thereby reducing scar tissue formation. What is your take on this?

This is a good question and it bears an intelligent response. The use of a Tuberculin Syringe to inject testosterone intramuscularly is not recommended (even though we do know many lean individuals doing it). These syringes are usually less than one half inch long and have a very narrow needle barrel. Injecting with such a small 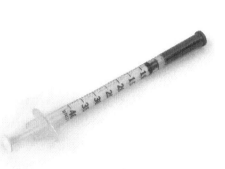 needle poses health risks. If a person is a newbie and does not possess low levels of body fat the chance at getting an infection at the point of injection exists. It is also extremely difficult to push the testosterone solution through the syringe when injecting due to the thinness of the needle.

MITIGATING AND AVOIDING POTENTIAL SIDE EFFECTS

CHAPTER 9

When undergoing TRT, it is IMPERATIVE your mindset is one of expecting and mitigating potential side effects. Sometimes the difference between successful lifelong TRT and crash-and-burn flameouts is both the patient and the TRT prescribing doctor knowing what to expect. As we age, our bodies change and often times quite rapidly. The side effects men may or may not experience are random and sometimes don't manifest for years if not decades.

It is crucially important to recognize the majority of potential side effects are minor and easily treatable. It is an unfortunate circumstance many men have received (and continue to receive) ineffective care from their TRT-prescribing physicians. Often times the inability to alleviate side effects forces men to end their treatment altogether. There is no reason for this whatsoever especially when you utilize the services of a progressive and experienced TRT prescribing physician.

http://TRTRev.com/trt-doctors

 As I have continued to stress throughout this book, it is CRUCIAL you keep detailed files on your blood panels in order to best understand your values as they change over time. Know thyself, compile blood panel data, and do your homework to ensure your TRT is successful over the long term. Become your own doctor. Study your reactions. Take notes. Be vigilant in knowing your body and what allows it to work optimally. Remember, doctors are said to have "practices" for a reason. They are human and do make mistakes.

You are the only one who truly knows your body, but only if you're paying attention.

Before discussing what I believe are the optimal ancillary medications, it's important to have a brief discussion on the primary issues and potential side effects men often face when undergoing TRT.

ESTRADIOL

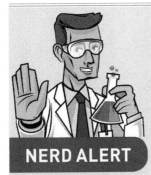

Estradiol monitoring and management is an important topic in TRT and recent studies have highlighted estradiol as just as important to male brain and sexual function as testosterone itself.87 Most of you know estrogen is the "female hormone" and what makes women "emotional". Actually estrogen is composed of three different forms, including one that plays a huge role in how men feel: estradiol (E2). So why is estradiol so important? It has profound implications for general health and has the potential to cause very unpleasant symptoms if levels are unbalanced. As testosterone levels decrease and estradiol levels increase, the ratio of free testosterone to estradiol reaches a critical point and estrogenic suppressive effects predominate.88

In my experience, both personally and in consulting with many men on TRT, the single biggest reason why TRT doesn't "work" is because of estradiol (E2) management. Usually it's out of balance. Unfortunately, a man can have side effects when suffering from low or high estradiol. From personal observation the single biggest determinant of whether estradiol (E2) is out of balance is erectile strength. Another obvious and noticeable side effect is water retention. Some men genetically overproduce aromatase which

---

87   Jankowska, E.A., Rozentryt, P., and Ponikowska, B. (2009). Circulating estradiol and mortality in men with systolic chronic heart failure. Journal of the American Medical Association. 2009 May 13;301(18):1892-901.

88   The role of estradiol in the maintenance of secondary hypogonadism in males in erectile dysfunction Cohen, P.G.Medical Hypotheses , Volume 50 , Issue 4 , 331 – 333

ultimately leads to increased estrogen production and its potential side effects. This is discussed in further detail later in this chapter.

It is of paramount importance to work with a knowledgeable TRT prescribing physician so both of you can dial in your estradiol from the start. Normally it will take an initial baseline blood estradiol (known as E2) panel and then future readings after starting TRT to figure out what level is best for the patient. There is a narrow therapeutic window regarding estradiol/estrogen where it is important for both patient and doctor to understand the optimal estradiol value range. Most knowledgeable TRT physicians will specify a 'sensitive' or 'enhanced' estradiol assay after a patient initiates TRT. This often times is critically important because the standard estradiol test is designed for women and tends to greatly overestimate estrogen.

TESTOSTERONE   DHT

Testosterone is converted to DHT within the body

DHT

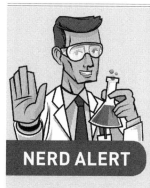

NERD ALERT

Even though the main androgen secreted by the testes is testosterone, the main androgenic signal comes from dihydrotestosterone (DHT). This includes the brain, central nervous system, skin and the genitals. Practically everything but muscle. Testosterone is converted to the active androgen DHT by the action of the enzyme 5 alpha reductase (5-AR). DHT because it binds about 3-5 times more strongly to the androgen receptor than testosterone, is much more anabolic in nature89.

89   Androgen receptor signaling induced by supraphysiological doses of dihydrotestosterone in human peripheral blood lymphocytes.Proteomics. 2010 Sep;10(17):3165-75.

DHT (dihydrotestosterone) is largely responsible for male pattern baldness. DHT can also cause benign growth of the prostate, increased oiliness of the skin and acne[90].

When you understand DHT in this fashion it is easy to believe your goal should be its elimination or reduction. But DHT is essential for proper brain chemistry and proper sexual function-including libido. Because of this odd duality, DHT is NOT something you want to reduce or eliminate in the body. But due to varying biochemical individuality, some men, will have to keep DHT levels under control as a prudent course of action. As always, great care and attention should be provided by your physician in monitoring your individual DHT levels relative to your initial baseline blood panel and ongoing blood panels over time. If you utilize TRT transdermally, it is very important to monitor your DHT levels as transdermals and creams often convert to DHT and will elevate PSA (prostate specific antigen) values transiently-usually until an effective dose of T is established.

PROLACTIN

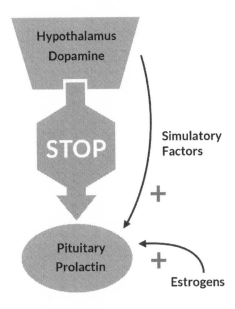

---

90   Dihydrotestosterone and the concept of 5alpha-reductase inhibition in human benign prostatic hyperplasia.Eur Urol. 2000 Apr;37(4):367-80.

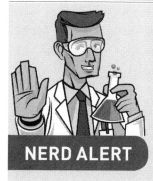

Prolactin is a hormone that can lower your testosterone and interfere with your sex life. Excessive prolactin is also associated with gynecomastia, i.e., "male boobs."[91] Studies have found high prolactin levels (known as hyperprolactinemia) in men are linked to low sexual desire and erectile dysfunction.[92] Men with severe hyperprolactinemia frequently show mild hypogonadism (low testosterone), and complain of a loss of libido and sexual dysfunction.[93]

NERD ALERT

If you are using TRT long term and start suffering a decline in libido, I encourage you to get your serum prolactin levels measured. A super high reading (> 300) may require your doctor to send for an MRI of the pituitary in case the issue is a pituitary adenoma. This is a non-cancerous pituitary tumor that can cause vision problems and headaches. It is either monitored (while tightly controlling estrogen and prolactin) or surgically removed through an amazingly routine procedure.

CAUTION

Many anti-aging clinics are using Cabergoline regularly in their practices with men to boost libido/and or improve sexual function[94]. Anecdotal studies show **one 0.5-milligram cabergoline tablet twice a week** improves the quality and intensity of sex drive, arousal, and orgasm. This is clearly an "off label" usage of this medication due to the lack of peer reviewed research data advocating it for this specific reason.

91   Bromocriptine monotherapy of a prolactinoma causing erectile dysfunction. Arch Esp Urol. 1997 Jun;50(5):526-8.

92   Hyperprolactinemia and Erectile Dysfunction. Rev Urol, 2000 Winter, 2(1):39–42,

93   Prolactin and testosterone: their role in male sexual function. Carani C1, Granata AR, Fustini MF, Marrama P.Int Androl.1996 Feb;19(1):48-54

94   Six months of treatment with cabergoline restores sexual potency in hyperprolactinemic males: an open longitudinal study monitoring nocturnal penile tumescence. J Clin Endocrinol Metab. 2004 Feb;89(2):621-5.

The author of this book has been prescribed and used almost every **SERM** (Selective Estrogen Receptor Modulator) and **AI**
(Aromatase Inhibitor) available.

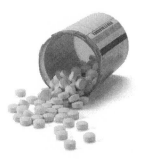

After many years of experience, I've cho-
sen (what I feel) are the OPTIMAL ancillary
medications for physicians to treat and safely correct potential TRT side effects. Some
men, due to the uniqueness of their biochemical individuality, will need
stronger side effect mediation than others.

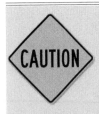

Because these **SERM's** and **AI's** have not been FDA
approved for use in males, TRT physicians prescribe them
'off-label'. Due to the fact that some of them are now
manufactured as generic medications in most markets, it
is unlikely a drug company would pursue FDA approval
for use in men now because of limited profit incentive,
mostly due to the relatively small market potential (for now at least). It is
important to understand these medications were designed to treat breast
cancer in women and as such they must be closely monitored when used in
male endocrine systems. They are usually well tolerated and a progressive
and experienced TRT physician should be quite familiar with their pharma
dynamics.

A progressive TRT-prescribing doctor will analyze your
lab work and symptoms and prescribe you ancillary
medications recommended in the chart below (when your
symptoms and/or blood values warrant it necessary) and will
discuss these potential side effects and their ramifications beforehand. This
will make them easier to identify for both of you. It is even more important
you are also learned in understanding and dealing with them as well. Again,
do your homework and know thyself.

Drug Classification	Name of Drug	Normal Dosage and Side Effects Addressed
SERM (Selective Estrogen Receptor Modulator)	Nolvadex (Tamoxifen) 10–20 mg Tablet	Nolvadex actually has quite a few applications for TRT users. First and foremost, its most common use is for the prevention of gynecomastia or male breast tissue growth otherwise known in locker room culture as "bitch tits". Nolvadex binds to the receptor site in breast tissue, safely preventing estrogen formation. The advantage of Nolvadex is it doesn't reduce estrogen in your body keeping some estrogen floating around. Estrogen is important for a properly functioning immune system and healthy joints. It has also been shown to improve lipid profiles (HDL and LDL) while using testosterone. [1]Normal dosage of Nolvadex is 10 mgs up to 40 mgs per day or EOD until symptoms disappear. Most progressive TRT physicians will taper the medication.

| SERM (Selective Estrogen Receptor Modulator) | Clomid (Clomiphene Citrate or Omifin) | Clomid works by blocking estrogen (E) action in the pituitary.[2] The pituitary thereby sees less estrogen and makes more luteinizing hormone (LH) due to removal of negative feedback inhibition. Increased LH levels in turn stimulate the Leydig cells in the testis to synthesize more testosterone. Clomid binds to estrogen receptors and also restores the body's natural production of testosterone[3]. Clomid is now preferred by a number of TRT Physicians like Jeffrey Dach MD[4], John Crisler DO[5], and Dr. Eugene Shippen[6] to be the preferential SERM used as 'mono-therapy' for hypogonadal men looking to remain fertile (retain motile sperm). These doctors have had great results using Clomid at 12.5 to 25 mgs EOD (every other day) to restore normal T production. In some men however, clomid increases SHBG which ultimately decreases free testosterone. As always careful evaluation of blood work is paramount. |

| SERM (Selective Estrogen Receptor Modulator) | Toremifene Citrate (Fareston) 60 mg Tablet | Toremifene while chemically similar to Nolvadex has several other well-known effects including acting as an estrogen antagonist in the hypothalamus and pituitary (HTPA). Because its androgenicity to estrogenicity ratio is 5x that of Nolvadex, toremifene is highly likely to be capable of increasing testosterone.[7] I find Toremifene as a good adjunct to dose with after long periods of TRT usage where an increase in libido is needed. It has been known to deliver a jolt to your HPTA improving sexual desire and intimacy feelings. A dosage of 30 mgs (half a tab) for two to three days in a row until libido and feelings of sexual desire are restored has been effective for some patients. This is another SERM rarely prescribed by TRT doctors. |

SERM (Selective Estrogen Receptor Modulator)	Raloxifene (Evista) 60 mg Tablet	Raloxifene is the newest SERM at the disposal of TRT physicians and their patients. Raloxifene is in the same family of compounds as Tamoxifen. Raloxifene has about 10x the binding affinity for the estrogen receptor in breast tissue than Tamoxifen[8]. It binds much more strongly to the receptor site, virtually eliminating the possibility of any estrogen reaching a receptor and exerting the undesired effect[9]. If you're reading between the lines, you can see how effective Raloxifene might be in the treatment and prevention of gynecomastia. An optimal dosing protocol is 60 mgs daily until gyno is gone.

| AI's (Aromatase Inhibitors) | Arimidex (Anastrozole) Tablet 1 mg Tablet | Arimidex is considered a "competitive inhibitor" AI which means it competes with estrogen around the aromatase enzyme. Arimidex performs by actively blocking the aromatase enzyme which inhibits the body's ability to produce estrogen. It is the most often doctor prescribed aromatase inhibitor (AI) due to its wide availability and effectiveness. An optimal dosing protocol of Arimidex while on TRT is 0.5 mg between once and 3 days a week. Some men will need to go as high as 1 mg EOD in order to prevent side effects such as moodiness, water retention and lowered libido. I feel men with higher body fat percentages will need 0.5 mg of Arimidex EOD when starting TRT as a good failsafe to prevent estrogenic side effects caused by elevated aromatase enzymes found in fat tissue. Arimidex does have the ability to reduce HDL cholesterol levels and needs to be monitored for this reason[10] |

AI's (Aromatase Inhibitors)	Aromasin (Exemestane) 25 mg Tablets	Aromasin is considered a "suicide inhibitor" AI which means it attaches to the aromatase enzyme and permanently disables it. Aromasin at 12.5–25 mgs a day, will raise testosterone levels by about 60%, and also help the free-to-bound testosterone ratio by lowering levels of sex hormone-binding globulin (SHBG) by 20%[11]. It's also highly compatible with Nolvadex and has beneficial effects on bone mineral content and lipid profiles. It suppresses estrogen more strongly than Arimidex but as a Type 1 inhibiting AI, once it deactivates the aromatase enzyme, it is rendered inactive allowing other ancillaries to continue to work.[12] This medication is widely misunderstood and it's rare for TRT physicians to prescribe it. It needs to be studied more closely due to its unique ability to raise testosterone levels via its reduction of SHBG.

AI's (Aromatase Inhibitors)	AIFM	AIFM[13] is an over-the-counter transdermal aromatase inhibitor that uses ATD, a natural steroidal aromatase inhibitor. Tested clinically in numerous animal and cell models, it is as effective as Aromasin but is not particularly well suited for oral administration as it has poor oral bioavailability.[14] Men can apply 1–3 pumps (200 to 600 mcl) twice a day to clean dry skin. 1–2 pumps to reduce moderate to high estrogen and 3 pumps for very high estrogen levels. You can apply it to inside of wrists and forearms, top of feet and upper vascular part of thigh/hip. I have known men to use it directly on sensitive excess estrogenic fat tissue around the breast/nipple area with good results. Even though this AI is not a pharmaceutical preparation, the active ingredient ATD is a pharmaceutical agent—just not scheduled/controlled by the DEA. It's one of those loophole agents classified as a nutritional supplement rather than an aromatase inhibitor. I have used this product in the past and received estrogen suppression similar to that of Arimidex.

TABLE FOOTNOTES

1   Furr BJ, Jordan VC (1984). "The pharmacology and clinical uses of tamoxifen". Pharmacol. Ther. 25 (2): 127–205. doi:10.1016/0163-7258(84)90043-3

2   Kim, E.D., et al., The treatment of hypogonadism in men of reproductive age. Fertil Steril, 2013. 99(3): p. 718-24.

3   Tan, RS; Vasudevan, D. (Jan 2003). "Use of clomiphene citrate to reverse premature andropause secondary to steroid abuse". Fertil Steril 79 (1): 203–5.

4   http://trtrev.com/dach

5   http://trtrev.com/crisler

6   http://trtrev.com/shippen

7   Price N, Sartor O, Hutson T, Mariani S. Role of 5a-reductase inhibitors and selective estrogen receptor modulators as potential chemopreventive agents for prostate cancer. Clin Prostate Cancer 2005;3:211-4. PMID 15882476

8   J Pediatr. 2004 Jul;145(1):71-6. Beneficial effects of raloxifene and tamoxifen in the treatment of pubertal gynecomastia.Lawrence SE, Faught KA, Vethamuthu J, Lawson ML.SourceDepartment of Pediatrics, University of Ottawa, Ontario, Canada.

9   Vogel, Victor; Joseph Constantino, Lawrence Wickerman et al. (2006-06-21). "Effects of Tamoxifen vs. Raloxifene on the Risk of Developing Invasive Breast Cancer and Other Disease Outcomes". The Journal of the American Medical Association 295 (23)

10   Rubinow KB, Tang C, Hoofnagle AN, et al. Acute Sex Steroid Withdrawal Increases Cholesterol Efflux Capacity and HDL-Associated Clusterin in Men.Steroids 2012;77(5):454-460. doi:10.1016/j.steroids.2012.01.002.

11   De Ronde W, de Jong FH. Aromatase inhibitors in men: effects and therapeutic options. Reproductive Biology and Endocrinology : RB&E 2011;9:93. doi:10.1186/1477-7827-9-93.

12   Simpson ER (2003). "Sources of estrogen and their importance". The Journal of Steroid Biochemistry and Molecular Biology 86 (3–5): 225–30. doi:10.1016/S0960-0760(03)00360-1. PMID 14623515

13   http://www.theafstore.com/product.php?productid=8&cat=0&page=&featured=Y

14   Steel E, Hutchinson JB. The aromatase inhibitor, 1,4,6-androstatriene-3,17-dione (ATD) blocks testosterone-induced olfactory behavior in the hamster. Cancer Res. 1981 Aug;42(8 Suppl): 3327s-3333s.

THE USAGE OF AROMATASE INHIBITORS (AI's) AND SELECTIVE ESTROGEN RECEPTOR MODULATORS (SERM's) AS TESTOSTERONE REPLACEMENT THERAPY (TRT)

It is becoming more commonplace for physicians to use a **SERM** (*selective estrogen receptor modulator*) such as *Clomid*, *Nolvadex* or *Toremifene*, or even an **AI** (*aromatase inhibitor*), such as *Arimidex*, as sole "TRT". These medications will elevate luteinizing hormone (LH) and overall total testosterone levels.[95] In my experience however, patients rarely report long term noticeable benefits (increased lean body mass, libido, less fatigue, etc.) from these strategies for the following reasons:

1. A major risk of using an AI alone is driving estrogen levels too low with potential deleterious consequences for the lipid profile, bone mineral density, libido, etc.

2. There is also a very narrow therapeutic window in regulating estrogen and estradiol levels that will impact on health and libido. Less, in terms of estrogen, is not necessarily better and these values need to be monitored on a regular basis with an experienced TRT physician. Remember, it is all about balance for the individual patient.

If your doctor has you on a SERM or AI as a form of TRT, we encourage you to show them this book so they can better understand why the usage of testosterone is much more effective strategy. Often times the usage of TRT however, will need to be combined with a SERM to achieve balance (between T and E) for the individual patient. **The noticeable exception is for younger TRT patients (30-50 years old) desiring to retain fertility**. These patients (as written more than once in this book) should ONLY consider using clomid or hCG monotherapy to help restore and improve low natural T production.

---

95   Short-term aromatase-enzyme blockade unmasks impaired feedback adaptations in luteinizing hormone and testosterone secretion in older men. Veldhuis JD1, Iranmanesh A. J Clin Endocrinol Metab. 2005 Jan;90(1):211-8. Epub 2004 Oct 13.

TRT protocols are inaccurate when AI's and SERM's are dosed without any corresponding elevated blood values or noticeable symptoms to indicate the patient needs either medication. There are *sometimes* exceptions to this rule. **Older men (usually over 50) and men with high body fat percentages** (for reasons previously discussed) can reasonably start a TRT protocol with an **AI** such as *Arimidex dosed at 0.5 mgs every other day* (EOD). After 21-30 days, if a patient starts to exhibit symptoms of unbalanced T and E, prescribing a SERM or modulating the therapeutic dosage of an AI is warranted until balance is achieved. And obviously vigilant observation of further lab work is necessary.

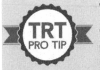

There are no hard and fast rules in regard to dosing the *aromatase inhibitors* (**AI's**) and *selective estrogen receptor modulators* (**SERM's**) medications. The dosing of these medications is highly variable. All men are biochemically different and why it is crucial to have a competent TRT prescribing doctor who can evaluate lab assays and attend to symptoms when the need arises. Again, ongoing and regular blood draws and patient feedback are crucial for both patient and doctor to achieve and maintain balance. With some men, balance can take time to achieve.

METABOLIC SYNDROME, OBESITY, AROMATASE AND ESTROGEN

Testosterone levels are lower in men with obesity, metabolic syndrome and type 2 diabetes[96]. As evidenced by just looking around, obesity is increasing at dramatic rates in most of the Western and Non-Western world. We all know the reasons. Poor diet, and a lack of exercise are the chief culprits.

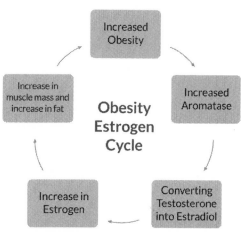

Recent studies indicate TRT in men with type 2 diabetes has beneficial effects on insulin resistance and visceral adiposity[97]. Most clinicians are aware insulin resistance and visceral fat play a key role in cardiovascular disease.

Testosterone replacement therapy has recently been proven to increase lean body mass (LBM), reduce fat mass and produce sustained and significant weight loss, reduction in waist circumference and BMI[98]. Wouldn't TRT in obese men with testosterone deficiency be a unique and effective therapeutic approach to the management of obesity? Of course it would.

Wouldn't it also make a lot of theoretical sense for men with type 2 diabetes and metabolic syndrome to consider having their testosterone levels measured? If found to be low or low normal, wouldn't a well designed TRT protocol (along with a proper diet and exercise program fully structured to reduce body fat) offer a reasonable strategy to optimize their health? Absolutely.

96   Wang C, Jackson G, Jones TH, et al. Low Testosterone Associated With Obesity and the Metabolic Syndrome Contributes to Sexual Dysfunction and Cardiovascular Disease Risk in Men With Type 2 Diabetes. Diabetes Care2011;34(7):1669-1675. doi:10.2337/dc10-2339.

97   Jones TH, Arver S, Behre HM, et al., TIMES2 Investigators. Testosterone Replacement in Hypogonadal Men With Type 2 Diabetes and/or Metabolic Syndrome (the TIMES2 Study). Diabetes Care 2011;34(4):828-837. doi:10.2337/dc10-1233.

98   Traish AM. Testosterone and weight loss: the evidence. Current Opinion in Endocrinology, Diabetes, and Obesity 2014;21(5):313-322. doi:10.1097/MED.0000000000000086.

Obesity
medical complications

PULMONARY DISEASE
abnormal function
obstructive sleep apnea
hypoventilation syndrome

IDIOPATHIC INTRACRANIAL
HYPERTENSION

STROKE

CATARACTS

NONALCOHOLIC
FATTY LIVER DISEASE
steatosis
steatohepatitis
cirrhosis

CORONARY
HEART DISEASE

← DIABETES

← DYSLIPIDEMIA

← HYPERTENSION

GALL BLADDER
DISEASE

SEVERE
PANCREATITIS

GYNECOLOGIC
ABNORMALITIES
abnormal menses
infertility
polycystic ovarian syndrome

CANCER
breast, uterus, cervix,
colon, esophagus, pancreas,
kidney, prostate,

OSTEOARTHRITIS

PHLEBITIS
venous stasis

SKIN

GOUT

Aromatase (as previously discussed) is more abundant in fat tissue.[99] The higher your body fat percentage, the more Aromatase enzymes floating around and the more likely you are to convert supplemental

---

99   The hypogonadal–obesity cycle: role of aromatase in modulating the testosterone–estradiol shunt – a major factor in the genesis of morbid obesity Cohen, P.G. Medical Hypotheses , Volume 52 , Issue 1 , 49 – 51

testosterone into estradiol (E2). Especially in the stubborn body fat[100] depot areas (Alpha Type 2A receptors) like the fat tissue found in the love handles, chest, and upper and lower back.

In other words, the higher your body fat percentage, the more likely you are to be susceptible to estradiol conversion and negative estrogenic side effects like moodiness, water retention, increased fat deposition, etc. A prudent course of action for high body fat percentage men starting TRT is to be put on a low dose AI like *Arimidex* to minimize the estrogen issues likely to arise.

*If your **body fat is above 20%**, (and to make every effort to minimize potential aromatization and estrogenic side effects) you should prioritize losing body fat[101] while undergoing TRT. I discuss strategies to optimize your fitness while on TRT in Chapter 12.*

---

100   http://fabfitover40.com/2014/03/09/struggle-removing-stubborn-body-fat/

101   http://fabfitover40.com/2014/01/01/tmcs-master-series-on-dieting-part-1-the-practical-approach/

CHAPTER 9 READER QUESTIONS

I'll appreciate any advice. Curiosity led to blood work, which revealed:

Test total: 156 (late afternoon test) Test free: 5.7, LH: 4.4, FSH: 2.6

I'm 32, and obese, 5'7 285. I've always been heavy set dude but these past three years were stupid, 60+ pounds gained. I'm seeing an endocrinologist in a few days but I don't expect much. What are the options? What should I read up on? I'd still like to have kids.

Thank you.

Being FAT (obese) will limit your body's ability to receive optimal results while using TRT. Too many men think they can live a FAT lifestyle and use TRT and get good results.

ABSOLUTELY NOT. Testosterone is not a panacea. It is an adjunct. A bump that helps people who have their diet and exercise already dialed in to improve a great many things (this book has already explained them). Using TRT when you are obese will most likely lead to issues with aromatase enzyme-ultimately leading to high E2 readings (estradiol), which WILL cause negative estrogenic side effects.

A good TRT dispensing doctor will NOT have any man in the 30-50 age range start a course of TRT (not until they have properly explored your ability to produce your own) if your #1 desire is having children. This physician should start you on a course of either *hCG* or Clomid monotherapy. Both of these medications will stimulate your leydig cells to increase Testosterone production via Luteinizing Hormone (LH) while also allowing you to remain fertile.

DO YOU HAVE ANY QUESTIONS ABOUT YOUR SPECIFIC SITUATION?

Just contact us by visiting this website:
http://TRTRev.com/questions

MONITORING TRT FOR OPTIMUM HEALTH

CHAPTER 10

If your goal is lifelong TRT administration (if this book has taught you anything, it should be) your vision and vigilance regarding monitoring your blood work should now begin in earnest. It is also of crucial importance to work with a TRT-prescribing physician who genuinely has your long-term goal of optimal health and safety at heart. It is also imperative you familiarize yourself with the following biomarkers and how they may be impacted by lifelong TRT administration. You should become acutely aware and educated on each so both you and your doctor can minimize or avoid issues before they arise. Taking any medication can adversely impact one's body chemistry and ignoring it is not advisable.

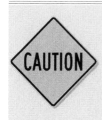

There is no reason to become overly paranoid or concerned about monitoring your blood work. A good TRT physician should alleviate most if not all of your worries. It is their job to observe and act when necessary. For those of you living where it is legal to be your own doctor, you must research and become intimately aware of your body's individual biochemical response to TRT.

UNDERSTANDING YOUR BLOOD PANELS AND LAB ASSAYS

After gathering your medical history, an informed TRT-prescribing physician will measure your blood work by running the following critically important assays.

- **Testosterone, Free and Total**
- **CBC specifically Hemoglobin/Hematocrit**
- **Sex Hormone Binding Globulin (SHBG)**
- **Homocysteine**
- **Estradiol (Sensitive or Enhanced)**
- **Vitamin D, 25-Hydroxy**
- **Prolactin**
- **C-Reactive Protein Quant**
- **Thyroid Panel**
- **Basic Metabolic Panel**
- **Lipid Panel**
- **DHEA-S**
- **Prostate Specific Ag Serum**

While all of them are important to monitor for out-of-range values, I'm going to focus on what I believe are the assays TRT users MUST keep a watchful eye on for the entire duration (ie lifelong) of their therapy.

Remember my recommendations in Chapter 4. In fact they are so important and relevant to this chapter--they bear repeating:

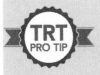

For *men in their 20's and 30's* fortunate enough to be undergoing TRT, I recommend you get your blood drawn *at least once a year.* For those of you in your *40's and up, twice a year is best.* An Anti-Aging Panel is highly recommended for anybody 35 and up.

If you are not already doing so, you should begin regularly getting your blood work done so you can compile and reference all of your data for life.

Having a detailed timeline from your very first/initial blood testosterone panel will provide excellent comparison points as your values and biomarkers change over time. Obviously your physician will be documenting this but I also recommend you keeping copies of your blood panels yourself so you can become intimately aware of the changes you experience. Do your homework and know your body. Study your reactions and take crystal clear notes. You will save yourself a lot of time when conversing with your doctor if you can speak intelligently with him/her regarding your own body and its reactions to TRT.

EVALUATING BLOOD TESTOSTERONE

Here is an actual excerpt from a blood test from a healthy and fit 33-year-old male with low body fat, who shockingly still suffers from low testosterone levels.

TESTS	RESULT	FLAG	UNITS	REFERENCE INTERVAL	LAB
CBC With Differential/Platelet					
WBC	4.5		x10E3/uL	3.4 - 10.8	01
RBC	4.61		x10E6/uL	4.14 - 5.80	01
Hemoglobin	14.6		g/dL	12.6 - 17.7	01
Hematocrit	44.6		%	37.5 - 51.0	01
MCV	97		fL	79 - 97	01
MCH	31.7		pg	26.6 - 33.0	01
MCHC	32.7		g/dL	31.5 - 35.7	01
RDW	13.6		%	12.3 - 15.4	01
Platelets	211		x10E3/uL	150 - 379	01
Neutrophils	50		%		01
Lymphs	39		%		01
Monocytes	7		%		01
Eos	3		%		01
Basos	1		%		01
Neutrophils (Absolute)	2.3		x10E3/uL	1.4 - 7.0	01
Lymphs (Absolute)	1.7		x10E3/uL	0.7 - 3.1	01
Monocytes(Absolute)	0.3		x10E3/uL	0.1 - 0.9	01
Eos (Absolute)	0.1		x10E3/uL	0.0 - 0.4	01
Baso (Absolute)	0.0		x10E3/uL	0.0 - 0.2	01
Immature Granulocytes	0		%		01
Immature Grans (Abs)	0.0		x10E3/uL	0.0 - 0.1	01
Testosterone,Free and Total					
Testosterone, Serum	**332**	**Low**	ng/dL	348 - 1197	01
Comment:					
Adult male reference interval is based on a population of lean males up to 40 years old.					
Free Testosterone(Direct)	**7.4**	**Low**	pg/mL	8.7 - 25.1	02
Prostate-Specific Ag, Serum					
Prostate Specific Ag, Serum	0.9		ng/mL	0.0 - 4.0	01
Roche ECLIA methodology.					
According to the American Urological Association, Serum PSA should					

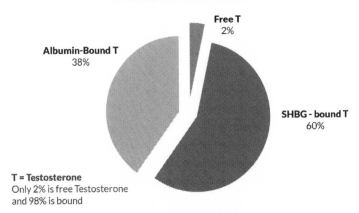

TESTOSTERONE FRACTIONS IN THE BLOOD

Free T
2%

Albumin-Bound T
38%

SHBG - bound T
60%

T = Testosterone
Only 2% is free Testosterone
and 98% is bound

Remember from Chapter 4 total testosterone is the concentration of testosterone in your blood stream and *free testosterone* is the small amount of testosterone floating around. Usually, only about 2% of the testosterone found in the body at any one time is 'free/active'[102] and *bio-available testosterone* (*BioT*) is 'active' or available for your body to use. Although the scales vary, testosterone levels are generally in a range of around **348 to 1197**—that's nanograms of testosterone per deciliter of blood per LabCorp. The scale varies depending on the blood laboratory performing the tests and the range is wide. Beyond drawing blood, there is no biochemical test administrable which can precisely measure between normal and abnormal levels of blood testosterone. Also age-specific ranges are not quoted because the values remain unclear. And remember the measurement is only of the particular time the sample was drawn. Think of it as snapshot of an extremely dynamic hormonal environment.

In the example above, the subject is out of range and low on testosterone. But what if someone is still within the range, but on the low end or middle part of the range (something like 400–600)? The problem with the scale is that it's **not adjusted for age**. Hence you could be 30 years old with testosterone levels of 300. That's normal—for a 70-year-old man. But isn't a 30 year old with the levels of a 70-year-old man running on empty? I argue definitively yes!

---

102   54. Vermeulen A, Verdonck L, Kaufman JM. A critical evaluation of simple methods for the estimation of free testosterone in serum. J Clin Endocrinol Metab.1999;84:3666–3672. [PubMed]

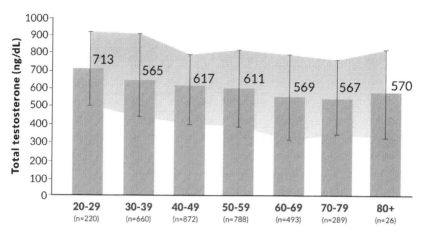

Also, the scale is based on percentiles. Let's say 225–348 ng/dl is the bottom 10th percentile and 1197 ng/dl is the top 10th percentile. At the 11th percentile, you're normal. But that's still significantly lower than what is nevertheless physiologically normal and attainable in 89% of other men. So even if you're technically "within range," you're not operating at optimal T levels for performance and well-being. And unfortunately many doctors won't prescribe their patients testosterone unless the patient is technically out-of-range. This means you could be 35 with T levels "within range" of an 80-year-old, but low for your age. This is again a reminder of why it is imperative for progressive TRT physicians to strive to treat the actual symptoms of their patients and not the findings of a lab report.

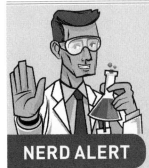

NERD ALERT

In a healthy young male, 60% of testosterone is attached to Sex Hormone-Binding Globulin (SHBG).[103] SHBG is produced mainly by the liver and then released into the bloodstream. Hormones bound to SHBG can't be used by the body and lose their anabolic effect. As men age, SHBG levels rise and bind strongly to the testosterone molecule lowering the body's absorption of free testosterone and its many benefits.[104] Hence, we want to have as much FREE (usable) testosterone available as possible. SHBG is an important marker of insulin resistance and studies have shown it an independent predictor of metabolic syndrome and type 2 diabetes[105]. In aging men, the rise in SHBG and associated maintenance of total testosterone values may mask low levels of free testosterone. SHBG is a critical component of proper TRT evaluation. It is imperative your doctor is vigilant to your SHBG and free testosterone levels while on TRT.

As just stated, Sex Hormone Binding Globulin (**SHBG**) is the fountainhead of proper hormonal evaluation. There are efficient ways to minimize the effects of **SHBG** and actually reduce its formation in the blood. Nettle root extract or Stinging Nettle Root[106] will lower SHBG ultimately increasing free testosterone[107]. Stinging Nettle Root also helps boost T levels by preventing its conversion to dihydrotestosterone (DHT). In fact, this author believes this supplement is a MUST HAVE for any man looking to make TRT a life long commitment. I recommend a divided dosage of ***750-1000 mgs per day*** preferably on

---

103   Hammond GL (2011). "Diverse Roles for Sex Hormone-Binding Globulin in Reproduction". Biology of Reproduction 85 (3): 431–441. doi:10.1095/biolreprod.111.092593. ISSN 0006-3363. PMID 21613632.

104   56 Diabetes Care. May 2004 v27 i5 p1036(6), "Testosterone and sex hormone-binding globulin predict the metabolic syndrome and diabetes in middle-aged men"

105   Stanworth RD, Jones TH. Testosterone for the aging male; current evidence and recommended practice . Clinical Interventions in Aging 2008;3(1):25-44.

106   http://trtrev.com/nettle

107   Lignans from the roots of Urtica dioica and their metabolites bind to human sex hormone binding globulin (SHBG). Planta Med. (1997)

an empty stomach. Dr. John Crisler also uses ***Danazol*** orally at 50 mg daily in select patients to lower SHBG[108].

HEMOGLOBIN AND HEMATOCRIT

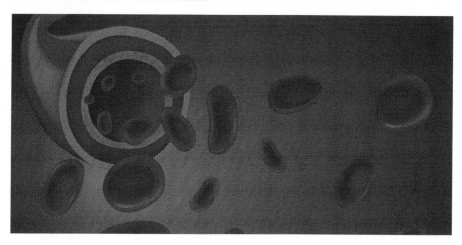

There is a noticeable correlation between high testosterone levels and high hemoglobin, most likely because testosterone stimulates increased red blood cell formation.[109] This increased production of RBC's (red blood cells) is called Erythrocytosis. Sometimes too many red blood cells causes polycythemia (blood thickening) which often develops during TRT in older men treated by injectable testosterone preparations.[110] They must get regular blood draws to siphon the excess RBC's. Depending on your age, the big picture is knowing hematocrit is a biomarker to become keenly aware of.

---

108   Testosterone Replacement Therapy-A Recipe for Success-Dr. John Crisler pg.33 Milestones Publishing (March 13, 2015)

109   Wang C, Nieschlag E, Swerdloff R, et al. Investigation, treatment and monitoring of late-onset hypogonadism in males: ISA, ISSAM, EAU, EAA and ASA recommendations.Eur J Endocrinol. 2008;159:507–514

110   Testosterone induces erythrocytosis via increased erythropoietin and suppressed hepcidin: evidence for a new erythropoietin/hemoglobin set point. Bhasin S4. J Gerontol A Biol Sci Med Sci. 2014 Jun;69(6):725-35. doi: 1093/gerona/glt154. Epub 2013 Oct 24.

Upon initial use of TRT, it is mandatory your physician monitors your hemoglobin/hematocrit levels vigilantly to make sure they stay under the range of *18 (Hemoglobin)/50 (Hematocrit)*. If they are elevated above these reference ranges, the periodic giving of blood (phlebotomy) should lower the value and function to keep it within range.[111] At my optimal dosage level of TRT, it is rare to have chronically elevated values, but it is still a crucially important biomarker for you and your physician to be pro-actively aware of and to aggressively treat with phlebotomy. Working with a knowledgeable TRT physician would ensure this never becomes an issue. Here is a short video where Dr Justin Saya discusses how elevated red blood cells are managed in men on TRT: http://TRTRev.com/manage-red-blood

LIVER HEALTH

There have been no documented cases of benign or malignant hepatic tumors with injectable or transdermal TRT.[112] There have been observed liver issues with long-term oral formulations of testosterone like methyltestosterone.[113] After nearly 15 years of active physician-guided TRT, the author has never once had elevated liver panels. It is my opinion detrimental lifestyle habits like consuming alcohol and eating diets high in saturated fats stress your liver far more than TRT ever will.

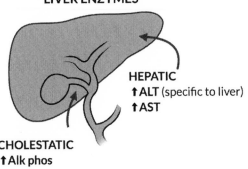

LIVER ENZYMES

HEPATIC
↑ ALT (specific to liver)
↑ AST

CHOLESTATIC
↑ Alk phos
↑ AAT

You should still have your liver enzymes measured once a year. If you experience any elevation I strongly encourage the supplement Tyler's

111   Nieschlag E. Testosterone treatment comes of age: new options for hypogonadal men. Clin Endocrinol (Oxf)2006;65:275–281. [PubMed

112   Gurakar A, Caraceni P, Fagiuoli S, Van Thiel DH. Androgenic/anabolic steroid-induced intrahepatic cholestasis: a review with four additional case reports. J Okla State Med Assoc.1994;87:399–404. [PubMed]

113   Westaby D, Ogle SJ, Paradinas FJ, Randell JB, Murray-Lyon IM. Liver damage from long-term methyltestosterone. Lancet.1977;2:262–263. [PubMed]

Liver Detox[114] to reduce risk and to lower elevated panel readings. (Also discussed in Chapter 11.)

PSA & Prostate Health

It is important to have a yearly PSA (prostate-specific antigen) screening while on TRT. Even with all the sensationalist claims in the media about how testosterone causes prostate cancer and benign prostatic hyperplasia (BPH) there is no conclusive evidence that TRT increases

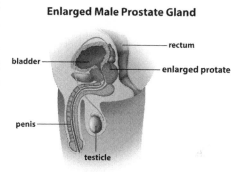

Enlarged Male Prostate Gland

rectum

bladder

enlarged protate

penis

testicle

the risk of prostate cancer or BPH.[115] In fact, in what I would call the *"Holy Grail of TRT and Prostate Cancer Research Data"* from Dr. R.M. Coward and Professor C.C. Carson[116] regarding the traditional model of testosterone-dependent prostate cancer growth (which suggested that greater serum testosterone concentrations would lead to greater cancer growth)—their recent findings appear to disprove the theory entirely.

---

114   http://trtrev.com/tyler

115   Marks LS, Mazer NA, Mostaghel E, et al. Effect of testosterone replacement therapy on prostate tissue in men with late-onset hypogonadism: a randomized controlled trial. JAMA. 2006;296:2351-2361.

116   http://www.trtrev.com/holy-grail-trt

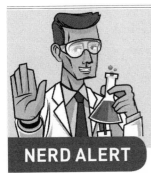

Rather, the most plausible explanation for what is seen clinically in the current era of TRT is supported by the recently re-evaluated saturation model, which states that, secondary to limited androgen receptor binding sites, prostate cancer growth is sensitive to variations in serum testosterone levels only below castrate range.[117]

NERD ALERT

Dr. Coward and Professor Carson go on to say the following:

"Based on all available data, as well as our personal experience, it is my opinion that testosterone deficiency syndrome can be safely treated with TRT after successful prostate cancer treatment."

In my opinion, this positive data has not gotten the exposure it deserves and more TRT-prescribing physicians should be aware of it. The Life Extension Foundation (LEF) citing Abraham Morgentaler, MD, in his landmark research article "Destroying the Myth About Testosterone Replacement and Prostate Cancer[118]" offers this positional stance on the risks of testosterone[119] and prostate cancer[120].

---

117   Morgentaler A, Traish AM. Shifting the paradigm of testosterone and prostate cancer: the saturation model and the limits of androgen-dependent growth. Eur Urol 2009;55:310–20

118   http://www.lef.org/magazine/2008/12/destroying-the-myth-about-testosterone-replacement-prostate-cancer/page-01

119   Morgentaler A. Testosterone and the prostate: is there really a problem? Contemporary Urol. 2006;18:26-33.

120   Testosterone and prostate safety. Front Horm Res. 2009;37:197-203. doi: 10.1159/000176054.

Low blood levels of testosterone do not protect against prostate cancer and, indeed, may increase the risk.

High blood levels of testosterone do not increase the risk of prostate cancer.

Treatment with testosterone does not increase the risk of prostate cancer, even among men who are already at high risk for it.

Clearly the paradigm is shifting as the medical community's knowledge of androgen physiology improves. This is awesome news and cause for celebration for male prostate cancer survivors the world over.

There is a possibility of TRT causing prostatitis or prostate infection/inflammation over long term use. While this is not dangerous, it can be troublesome causing restricted urine flow and frequent nighttime urination symptoms. There are a number of potential treatments to consider.

5-alpha reductase inhibitors such as **Flomax** or **Uroxatral** relax the smooth muscle of the prostate wall and bladder neck often improving urine flow[121]. A more radical but efficient approach is the use of a laser[122] to eliminate any prostate tissue obstruction.[123] PSA levels have been known to rise in older men at the start of transdermal T delivery systems due to them elevating DHT. Normally once testosterone levels have stabilized, PSA will drop back down into a baseline range.

Recently the usage of **Cialis[124] (Tadalafil)** (the erectile dysfunction drug) at 2.5 mgs to 5 mgs every day has also been approved for the treatment of BPH.[125]

121   The efficacy and safety of alpha-1 blockers for benign prostatic hyperplasia: an overview of 15 systematic review-J, Liu, Y, Yang Z, Qin X, Yang K, Mao C. Curr Med Res Opin. 2013 Mar;29(3):279-87.

122   http://www.amsgreenlight.com/HPS_intro.html

123   Photoselective laser vaporization of the prostate (PVP) for the treatment of benign prostatic hyperplasia (BPH): 12-month Results from the First United States Multi-center Prospective Trial. J Urol 2004; 172:1404-1408

124   http://trtrev.com/cialis

125   Latest pharmacotherapy options for benign prostatic hyperplasia. Expert Opin Pharmacother. 2014 Epub 2014 Aug 28th.

BLOOD PRESSURE

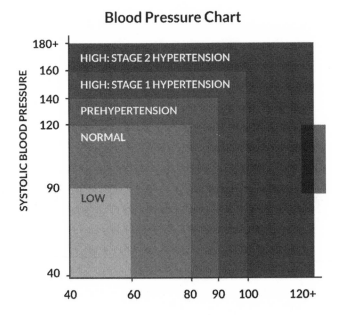

It is always important to monitor blood pressure (BP) as it remains the #1 "silent killer" in the world due to its ability to cause strokes and heart attacks. As I have previously stated throughout the book, unfortunately some men with higher body fat percentages convert testosterone into estradiol more readily. Some men also have genetically higher levels of aromatase enzymes[126] which will also negatively impact testosterone values.

High levels of estradiol can cause water retention which can lead to high blood pressure. Most of the studies indicate clinical TRT dosing protocols rarely affect blood pressure. You should get your BP measured in the first month of TRT just as a failsafe to see whether it's increasing over your normal baseline BP.

---

126   Czajka-Oraniec I, Simpson ER (2010). "Aromatase research and its clinical significance".Endokrynol Pol 61 (1): 126–34. PMID 20205115.

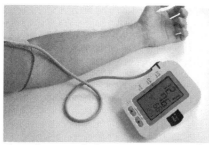

You can purchase a blood pressure cuff[127] over-the-counter and do it at home or you can choose to visit your local pharmacy to measure regularly (in addition to having it monitored with regular office visits to your physician). As already stated, become aware of your normal blood pressure values and understand when your readings are elevated.

Heart and Vascular Health

There is widespread misinformation that TRT increases the risk of vascular events or disease. You've probably seen or heard one of the many different multimedia ads about TRT causing heart issues. These ads claim if you've used TRT you may be entitled to a financial recovery. What can I say? We live in a very litigious society and the attorneys filing the lawsuits are opportunistic.

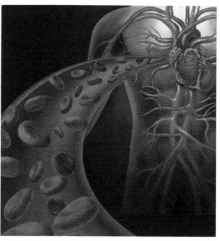

Based on the most recent research on the matter[128] and disputing the TOM[129] and JAMA[130] studies in question, there is NO EVIDENCE

---

127   http://trtrev.com/cuff

128   Patel P et al. Abstract 1195-376. Zuber A et al. Abstract 1126M-13. Both presented at: American College of Cardiology (ACC) 64th Annual Scientific Session & Expo; March 14-16, 2015; San Diego

129   Basaria S, Davda MN, Travison TG, Ulloor J, Singh R, Bhasin S. Risk Factors Associated With Cardiovascular Events During Testosterone Administration in Older Men With Mobility Limitation. The Journals of Gerontology Series A: Biological Sciences and Medical Sciences. 2013;68(2):153-160. doi:10.1093/gerona/gls 138.

130   Vigen R, O'Donnell, Baron AE, et al. Association of testosterone therapy with mortality, myocardial infarction, and stroke in men with low testosterone levels. JAMA 2013; 310:1829-1835.Cappola AR. Testosterone therapy and risk of cardiovascular disease in men. JAMA 2013; 310:1805-1806.

to support the statement 'TRT causes increased risk of heart attacks and strokes' in ***any man under the age of 65***.

If it were true, every teenager would have cancer and heart disease. (For more information disputing this study's data, see the interview with Dr. Brett Osborn[131] in Chapter 13).

In randomized placebo controlled trials, TRT *DOES NOT* increase the incidence of cardiovascular disease or events such as myocardial infarction, stroke, or angina.[132]

Older men often face an increased risk for vascular problems as in many other areas of their health. But there is no conclusive research available stating the risk of using TRT further endangers them beyond their normal increased risk. Most of the data available (and prior to these trolling class action cases coming to the foreground) provides clear evidence *supplemental testosterone reduces the risk of cardiovascular events in otherwise healthy and normal men*[133].

One other biomarker to be aware of as a potential vascular issue is **homocysteine**. Homocysteine is an amino acid when present in high concentrations, has been linked to an increased risk of heart attacks and strokes[134]. Observed normal levels of homocysteine are between 4.4 and 10.8 micromoles per liter of blood. Elevated **homocysteine levels** are thought to contribute to plaque formation by damaging arterial walls. I recommend supplementing with *B Complex*[135], *Folic Acid*[136] and *SAMe*[137] as excellent over the counter (OTC) supplements to reduce elevated levels. Additionally, an always prudent vascular protectant as we age is investing in regular and consistent endurance exercise. I discuss this much more in Chapter 12.

131   http://trtrev.com/osborn

132   Testosterone and cardiovascular risk in men: a systematic review and meta-analysis of randomized placebo-controlled trials. Mayo Clin Proc. 2007;82(1):11–13. [PubMed]

133   Oskui PM, French WJ, Herring MJ, Mayeda GS, Burstein S, Kloner RA. Testosterone and the Cardiovascular System: A Comprehensive Review of the Clinical Literature. Journal of the American Heart Association: Cardiovascular and Cerebrovascular Disease. 2013;2(6):e000272. doi:10.1161/JAHA.113.000272.

134   Correlation Between Hyperhomocysteinemia and Outcomes of Patients With Acute Myocardial Infarction. Am J Ther. 2014 Nov 17.

135   http://trtrev.com/b-complex

136   http://trtrev.com/folic-acid

137   http://trtrev.com/same

LIPIDS AND CHOLESTEROL HEALTH

TRT has been shown to have little to no effect on plasma HDL levels in multiple studies[138]. TRT has been shown to decrease triglycerides and LDL levels[139]. It's always important to have your low-density lipoprotein (LDL) and high-density lipoprotein (HDL) along with your triglycerides checked while in a fasted state at least once a year.

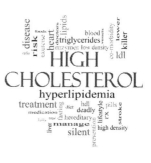

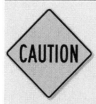

Many TRT-prescribing clinicians believe testosterone can negatively impact cholesterol levels. This belief is not supported by any relevant data. It is assumed the excessively high doses (supraphysiologic) of testosterone and other synthetics (anabolic steroids) used by athletes and pro/recreational bodybuilders leads to reductions in **HDL** (high-density lipoprotein a.k.a. the beneficial cholesterol) and increases in **LDL** (low-density lipoprotein a.k.a. the negative cholesterol). There is no conclusive peer-accepted research to support these beliefs—only the elevated cholesterol values seen in the private panels of these population groups.

---

138   Pharmacokinetics, efficacy, and safety of a permeation enhanced testosterone transdermal system in comparison with bi-weekly injections of testosterone enanthate for the treatment of hypogonadal men. J Clin Endocrinol Metab. 1999;84:3469–3478. [PubMed]

139   Chrysohoou C, Panagiotakos D, Pitsavos C, et al. Low Total Testosterone Levels are Associated With the Metabolic Syndrome in Elderly Men: The Role of Body Weight, Lipids, Insulin Resistance, and Inflammation; The Ikaria Study. The Review of Diabetic Studies : RDS 2013;10(1):27-38. doi:10.1900/RDS.2013.10.27.

Improving your cholesterol can be accomplished with diet and exercise modification. Proper eating and some form of exercise should be the established foundation prior to beginning any treatment. Chronically poor levels of cholesterol can increase your risk of cardiovascular disease. Sometimes medical intervention is needed to help restore a proper lipid balance. Here are three over the counter supplements which have shown to improve your lipid profile. Each nutrient works differently. 1) Omega-3 Fish Oil 2) Co-Q10 3) Red Yeast Rice.

Doctors sometimes prescribe Omega-3 as a blood thinner, found to be more effective than Asprin, for patients found to have high red blood cells. This can be especially beneficial to men on TRT

Statin Drugs are commonly prescribed by Doctors to patients who have high cholesterol. Nearly 60 million people will be taking statin drugs this year in the United States alone. Statins have been found to significantly lower Co-Q10 levels. Supplementing with Co-Q 10 can help restore depleted levels.

BALDNESS AND ACNE

Baldness, otherwise known as 'male pattern baldness' (**MPB**), is genetic. Using TRT can definitely exacerbate or speed up hair loss for those prone to it via testosterone converting into *dihydrotestosterone* (**DHT**). The idea of losing hair is very difficult to deal with for many men. I believe accepting symptoms of low testosterone in order to retain a receding or thinning hair line is an unequal trade off. In fact it is silly. Sometimes the difference between acting 'alpha' and living 'beta' is shaving your head in order to enjoy the myriad benefits higher testosterone provides.

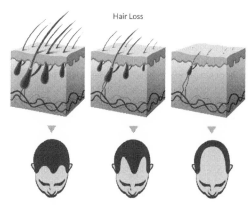

Hair Loss

There are numerous medications men take to prevent thinning hair from receding entirely. The most popular are **Propecia**[140] also known as **Proscar**. The active ingredient in Propecia is **Finasteride** which is a *5-alpha-reductase* (**5AR**) *inhibitor*. It works by blocking the enzymes that naturally convert testosterone into *dihydrotestosterone* (DHT). The problem with **5AR** inhibitors is not only do they inhibit the testosterone molecule itself (lessening many of the positive effects) it also reduces libido (sex drive) and weakens erections.[141] It also may reduce fertility and lower sperm count.[142] You want to experience this at the expense of keeping hair that is already falling out? No thanks, gentlemen. If your hair is that important to you, I recommend a topical application[143] to directly affect hair at the root and to learn more about hair loss causes and available topical treatments[144].

Dihydrotestosterone (**DHT**) is also known to have negative effects on the skin and hair follicles. **DHT** increases the production of oil in the sebaceous glands which often leads to

---

140   http://trtrev.com/propecia

141   The dark side of 5⊠-reductase inhibitors' therapy: sexual dysfunction, high Gleason grade prostate cancer and depression. Traish AM1, Mulgaonkar A2, Giordano N2. Korean J Urol. 2014 Jun;55(6):367-79. Epub 2014 Jun 16.

142   Finasteride and male infertility: a case for prospective collaborative research databases?
Fertility and Sterility, Volume 100, Issue 6, December 2013, Pages 1528-1529

143   http://www.excelmale.com/showthread.php?418-Hair-loss-remedies-while-on-trt& highlight=Topical+Hair+Loss+Solution

144   http://trtrev.com/hair-loss

bouts of acne. For those men who were prone to incidences of acne in their teen years, testosterone may or may not cause flare-ups on their backs and shoulders later.

It is my belief diet is often the source of acne. Eating a diet high in essential fatty acids (EFA's) along with reducing refined and processed food consumption can make a big difference in clearing up the oily skin that leads to acne. We discuss what constitutes a clean diet in Chapter 11. There is a genetic component to acne and some men may do well by consulting a dermatologist for severe issues. Dr Justin Saya discusses how to manage acne during TRT[145].

TESTICULAR SHRINKAGE, LOW SPERM COUNT AND HPTA/HPGA DYSFUNCTION

It is important to understand male reproduction and fertility is a highly inexact science. There are tremendous inter-individual differences in endocrinology, especially when it relates to the hypothalamus, pituitary and testes.[146] Supplemental testosterone inhibits the body's own (endogenous) production through negative feedback inhibition of *luteinizing hormone* (**LH**) levels. This results in suppression of *follicle-stimulating hormone* (**FSH**) levels which leads to suppression of sperm production (*azospermia*).

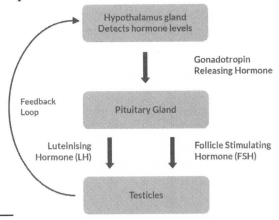

---

145   http://trtrev.com/acne

146   Crabbe, P., et al., Part of the interindividual variation in serum testosterone levels in healthy men reflects differences in androgen sensitivity and feedback set point: contribution of the androgen receptor polyglutamine tract polymorphism. J Clin Endocrinol Metab, 2007. 92(9): p. 3604-10

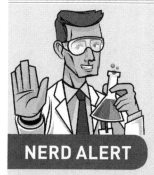

When exogenous (supplemental) testosterone is used, a cascade of biochemical actions take place. Your hypothalamus (the master gland in your brain) secretes **GnRH** (*Gonadotropin Releasing Hormone*), which causes your pituitary gland to secrete *luteinizing hormone* (**LH**) and *follicle-stimulating hormone* (**FSH**). The increase in these hormones causes the testes to stimulate the Leydig cells to produce testosterone (by conversion of cholesterol). Testosterone then has the ability to undergo various metabolic processes that will inhibit **GnRH**, which in turn inhibits the secretion of **LH** and **FSH**, bringing a halt to endogenous (natural) testosterone production. This is referred to as the *negative feedback loop*. Once testosterone has stopped being produced, it no longer sends this negative signal, and GnRH eventually begins to do its job again. This is how homeostasis is maintained in the human body.

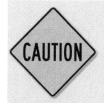

All men should be fully cognizant using lifelong TRT protocols (like those found in this book) can definitely (and most likely WILL) reduce the size of your testes, interfere with fertility and suppress your **HPTA** (*Hypothalamic-Pituitary-Testicular Axis*) also known as the **HPGA** (*Hypothalamic–Pituitary–Gonadal Axis*) and sometimes now known as the **HPG Axis**. This means your natural testosterone production will be impaired if not SHUT DOWN altogether. This is nothing to worry about whether you are past your reproductive age or not. This is tackled further in the reader question and answer section later in this chapter.

Based on my personal experiences using TRT and consulting with numerous men, there *are* solutions to maintaining fertility while using TRT. There are highly effective fertility medications (**hCG**, clomiphene citrate (**clomid**) and **hMG**) that, when administered by an experienced and knowledgeable TRT physician, will allow men to restore natural testosterone production ultimately leading to normal reproductive and sexual function[147].

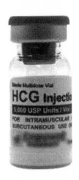

Using *human chorionic gonadotropin* (**hCG**)[148] every so often (daily, weekly to perhaps even every other week) at a dosage of ***250 to 500 iu's per injection*** (injecting subcutaneously into the fat tissue of lower stomach or the fat pad of outer glute with an insulin syringe) will provide your testicles an increase in size or fullness. **hCG** has been clinically proven to restore fertility in men undergoing TRT[149]. Some men psychologically need this cosmetic effect of full testicles to feel normal. The "John Crisler Method of hCG is injecting the last two days before a once a week T injection protocol or if injecting T twice weekly, injecting **hCG** on the day before each injection[150]. It is important to monitor **hCG** as it *CAN* elevate estradiol (E2) potentially causing estrogenic side effects in men with higher body fat percentages and higher genetic production of aromatase due to its ability to elevate aromatase enzymes.

For those of you wishing to retain your fertility, fret not. **Human menopausal gonadotropin (hMG)** is a potent female fertility medication which can also increase sperm count and stimulate sperm motility in men[151]. **hMG** is stronger than **hCG** because it mimics both **LH** and **FSH** and additionally binds to receptors in the testicles **hCG** alone will not bind to.[152]

147   Preserving fertility in the hypogonadal patient: an update. Asian J Androl. 2014 Oct 3. doi: 10.4103/1008-682X.142772. [Epub ahead of print]

148   http://trtrev.com/hcg

149   Ramasamy R, Stahl PJ, Schlegel PN. Medical therapy for spermatogenic failure. Asian Journal of Andrology 2012;14(1):57-60. doi:10.1038/aja.2011.63.

150   Testosterone Replacement Therapy-A Recipe for Success-Dr. John Crisler pg.73 Milestones Publishing (March 13, 2015)

151   Hwang K, Walters RC, Lipshultz LI. Contemporary concepts in the evaluation and management of male infertility. Nature reviews. Urology 2011;8(2):86-94. doi:10.1038/nrurol.2010.230.

152   Rate, extent, and modifiers of spermatogenic recovery after hormonal male contraception: an integrated analysis Lancet. 2006 Apr 29;367(9520):1412-20.

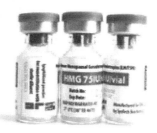

I have known men who were on TRT for many years straight and after using **hMG in combination with hCG** at a very minimum *dose of 0.75 iu's per day for 5–7 days in a row*, got their wives or girlfriends pregnant within one month of beginning administration. For any of you utilizing TRT and struggling to father children (just using hCG or Clomid) give this book to your physician so he is informed and aware of this highly effective **SERM**. For an excellent dosing strategy using *hCG* and *hMG* in combination, Web MD has an excellent article[153]. Dr. Justin Saya also has a good video explanation of hCG as well.[154]

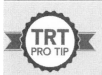

While some men are able to get a prescription for testosterone from their local primary care doctor, some often have trouble getting a prescription for ancillary medications including hCG. If that is the case and you want to consult with an experienced doctor, doing so via telemedicine by phone or webcam is a convenient alternative. If a prescription is written, medication can then be shipped directly to you from the pharmacy. This is a great service for men who do not have easy local access to TRT and related treatments. Visit this website to discover more: http://TRTRev.com/hcg

---

153   http://www.webmd.com/infertility-and-reproduction/gonadotropin-treatment-for-infertility

154   http://trtrev.com/hcg-video

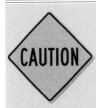

Some physicians prescribe **hCG** and/or **clomid monotherapy** as a form of TRT. The premise of this protocol is to stimulate the testicles with either **hCG or clomid** so they increase testosterone production. Its success rate is highly dependant on how sensitive the leydig cells are in the individual patient's testicles. This is the PREFERRED strategy for younger men (30-50 age group) desiring to maintain fertility and higher sperm count (who are *ATTEMPTING* to NOT DISRUPT their endogenous testosterone production). There is no peer reviewed research stating **hCG or clomid** *causes* or *does not cause* HPTA shutdown. Again it is important to monitor blood panels of E2 (estradiol) when on long term **hCG** or **clomid** therapy due to their potential to increase aromatase activity. As already stated in Chapter 9 there are highly successful TRT physicians using Clomid as their sole form of therapy to restore T production in hypogonadal men concerned with retaining their fertility.

I highly recommend *men still interested in maintaining their fertility* consider visiting their urologist and getting a **measured sperm count** in order to understand their baseline values before undergoing TRT. It would also be prudent to have sperm frozen to be used at a later date as a precautionary measure.

The myth propagated by the media about testosterone causing a man's penis to shrink is nonsense. If anything, the penis can increase in size and/or girth as testosterone increases nitric oxide production stimulating nitrogen retention, which enhances blood flow causing

harder and thicker erections.[155] Whether this is temporary due to increased nitric oxide synthase production is unknown.[156] It stands to reason if a man is on TRT for life, this temporary effect might appear more permanent.

---

155   Recent insights into androgen action on the anatomical and physiological substrate of penile erection. Asian J Androl. 2006;8:3–9. [PubMed] Gooren LJ, Saad F.

156   Investigation, treatment and monitoring of late-onset hypogonadism in males: ISA, ISSAM, EAU, EAA and ASA recommendations. Eur J Endocrinol.2008;159:507–514. Wang C, Nieschlag E, Swerdloff R, et al.

WHY CYCLING TESTOSTERONE IS INEFFECTIVE

Cycling on and off testosterone has no business being used in the therapeutic administration of TRT. The myriad benefits are so advantageous why would an aging man want to come off? It has been clearly proven men's natural testosterone declines by 1% (at the least) per year after the age of 30.[157] Choosing to use TRT to maintain optimum blood levels (sustainable with proper lab blood values) should be a lifelong commitment[158] regardless of age. The physicians who intermittently use **hCG** also use it as a "break" in TRT, much the same way hormonally-supplemented athletes manage typical anabolic steroid cycles. Again, TRT should not be "cycled". Many doctors erroneously believe 'cycling' allows the HPTA to recover. The **hCG**-induced testosterone production is sometimes every bit as suppressive of the **HPTA/HPGA** as the TRT itself. As to the argument some doctors make about 'cycling' to maintain spermatogenesis and avoid sterility—it has been proven supplementing with **hCG** and/or **hMG** (as previously written) while on TRT allows men to retain their fertility.[159]

The mindset of cycling was created by underground anabolic steroid dealers to sell more drugs necessary to medicate the side effects caused by high dosages of these synthetics, i.e. anabolic steroids. These side effects caused men to have severe endocrine system disruptions when going on and off (known as yo-yoing). Cycling as it's known had to happen because men using anabolics (synthetics) were often taking multiple drugs at once (known as stacking) in supraphysiologic doses putting their endocrine systems at risk. When using TRT under the guidance of an experienced and knowledgeable physician, optimal blood levels of testosterone are easily sustainable throughout an adult male's life. Again the TRT protocols discussed and recommended in this book are about HEALTH. PERIOD.

---

157   Morley JE, Perry HM 3rd: Androgen deficiency in aging men: role of testosterone replacement therapy. J Lab Clin Med 2000;135:370-378

158   http://trtrev.com/cycling

159   Authors: Rastrelli G, Corona G, Mannucci E, Maggi M Andrology. 2014 Oct 1; Factors affecting spermatogenesis upon gonadotropin-replacement therapy: a meta-analytic study

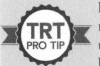 I can't stress enough how important it is for every man reading this book to take control of his health while undergoing TRT by regular and methodical collection of blood panels. Order the Hormone and Wellness Panel for Men[160] first and if you're already a lifelong TRT patient, get a couple of the TRT Male Hormone/Wellness Follow Up Panels[161] done per year. Be proactive always and take your health into your own hands.

---

160   http://trtrev.com/hormone-panel
161   http://trtrev.com/trt-hormone-panel

Here is a Chart or a Cheat Sheet for the most important biomarkers/lab assays for men to monitor regularly while undergoing lifelong TRT.

Test/Exam	Frequency/Where
Blood Pressure (especially if you have too much body fat)	*Weekly or semi-monthly* via purchase of an over-the-counter cuff, or at a pharmacy or an office visit with your physician.
CBC-Hemoglobin or **Hematocrit (H/H)**	*Twice during your first year on TRT, then annually.* Need to make sure numbers don't exceed 18 (Hemoglobin)/50 (Hematocrit). Any elevation beyond is an indication to donate blood (Phlebotomy) or possibly withhold TRT until RBC's (red blood cells) are increased. Some patients may need to be phlebotomized multiple times a year while undergoing testosterone replacement therapy.
Comprehensive Metabolic Panel	**Once a year.** Many strength trainers/weight lifters consume extra protein and supplements like Creatine which can create false positive elevations in Blood Urea Nitrogen (BUN) and Creatinine. An informed TRT physician will know to survey this in their patients and avoid suspecting kidney or liver problems.
Lipid Panels	*At least once a year via a fasted blood test.*
Prostate Specific Antigen (PSA) Value	*Baseline and then yearly* (consultation with physician for further details). When utilizing transdermal delivery systems, it is important to monitor this marker as DHT can increase PSA rapidly upon initiation of therapy.

Digital Rectal Exam (DRE)	*Once a year after age 45* (especially if family history).
Estradiol (E2)	*After a baseline is attained before and during TRT, 1-2x per year* to ensure proper balance dependent on side effects or symptoms. Best to order 'enhanced', 'sensitive', or 'ultra sensitive' to better evaluate male symptomatology regarding estrogen levels.
Prolactin	*After baseline is attained before and during TRT, 1x per year* based on perceived symptoms/side effects (such as a loss of libido or feelings of moodiness or depression). Elevated prolactin over 300 should result in an MRI checking for a pituitary adenoma.
C-Reactive Protein	*Once a year after age 40.*
Homocysteine	*2x a year.*
DHEA	*1x a year for men over 40.* Make sure to test DHEA-S as there is much more S in the body which provides more to measure. DHEA is a tricky hormone but it has a lot of potential life enhancing qualities. Read this amazing article about DHEA[15] and whether you should consider supplementing with it.

Chapter 10 Reader Questions

Do I have to be on TRT forever? Do you get permanently addicted?

Since your body will not produce the optimal levels of T by itself (upon long term lifelong TRT), you must continue TRT if you want to maintain the benefits. But why wouldn't you want to live a life filled with virility? No different than taking a bath/shower or eating food regularly. There is no such purpose for cycling when you're doing TRT correctly per my recommendations and as a lifelong pursuit.

Too many men get caught up in the mindset of "Oh no, if I stay on forever and lose my natural production, then what?" Well, you'll never have to worry about low testosterone and all the problems it causes because the truth is very simple and easy to face. If you don't make the choice to improve your declining natural production (total and free testosterone LESSENS every single day after the age of 30[162] and perhaps younger) with a replacement dose, you'll eventually experience the symptoms of suffering from lower testosterone.

Does TRT make me sterile and unable to have children?

This is a myth and untrue. If you desire to have children, make sure you also strategize the usage of either **hCG, clomid** and/or **hMG** in your usage of testosterone. As previously stated, you should also visit your urologist to get a **measured sperm count** in order to understand your baseline values before starting TRT. TRT usually will not permanently damage your ability to impregnate a woman. In the worst cases I have seen—where men who were on TRT for more than 10 years and were totally inhibited via luteinizing hormone (LH) and follicle stimulating hormone (FSH) values, using a rigorous course of **hCG** and/or clomid or **hMG** restored fertility within six months and sometimes in less time.

---

162   Morley JE, Perry HM 3rd: Androgen deficiency in aging men: role of testosterone replacement therapy. J Lab Clin Med 2000;135:370-378

With all the sensationalist claims in the news about testosterone increasing the possibility of CV (cardiovascular) events like heart attacks, strokes, etc., and your book clearly dispelling them as poorly and wrongly interpreted data from older men in higher risk population groups, what is the prudent course of action knowing there is NO CONCLUSIVE longer term studies proving the safety of TRT?

This a great question and one deserving of an elaborate answer.

Actually there is a myriad of studies documenting the SAFETY of T replacement (more so than those documenting the contrary). As with ANYTHING, precautions must be exercised (no pun intended) and T replacement should ONLY be pursued under the watchful eye of a knowledgeable and experienced TRT supervising physician. The benefits of T, as opposed to being wholly biochemical in nature, may be a function of the hormone's effect on fatigue, secondarily increasing one's tendency to exercise and pursue a more physical lifestyle. This by virtue confers protection AGAINST coronary disease. No one questions EXERCISE'S health improving effects, right?

Assuming the WORST, the data are mixed: 50/50. In our professional opinion however, considering that the HRT-associated "risk" is likely a function of flawed study design (and therefore spurious), it is WORTH the risk.

Hey Jay-Quick question

Background – I have had trouble finding a good TRT doc in Denver without spending upward of $3k just to get started. I paid for my own lab work, used the bloodwork video from you and put myself on TRT with black market test. So far everything has been great.

My real point – As any good doc knows, after a period of time on TRT one's natural production shuts off. Do you think/know of a Doctor who would work with me on this, without forcing me to go on a hormonal/emotional rollercoaster just to "prove" that my natural levels are crap ie crashing my current test levels just to qualify for legit TRT script?

This is also a great question. The Folks at Defy Medical provided me the best answer. You would not need to stop your hormone supplementation. On your initial panel they will detect you are taking an androgen. They will encourage you and all men in similar situations to be honest. If they know you are using testosterone, they will continue your TRT without disruption but will modify the protocol (dosage)l to get all numbers within a good range.

Defy's Doctors will want to know what you were using, how long, etc. If you are young, less than 35 years old, and only using underground AAS than the doctors will have you stop and do an HPTA stimulation protocol.

Nutrition and its Role in TRT
Chapter 11

In Chapters 11 and 12 I discuss optimizing your testosterone replacement therapy through correct nutrition and exercise. It is crucial to understand the powerful role diet and exercise play in the maintenance of TRT. You WILL improve results dramatically by ensuring diet and exercise strategies are dialed in. Dr. Brett Osborn's book GET SERIOUS[163] is highly recommended as an excellent resource guide for understanding the how and why of proper nutrition and exercise.

It's important we clarify some things for all men reading this book. If you are a man who drinks alcohol nightly and whose diet consists of fast food, sodas and other processed food, you will not experience the wonders of higher levels of testosterone. Testosterone WILL NEVER BE a magic bullet or panacea wonder supplement when used in combination with an unhealthy lifestyle. *If you eat a clean diet and use an intelligently-designed resistance and endurance training program while also being on a sound TRT regimen—your results should be outstanding.*

Let's first discuss how to best structure your diet and nutrition to maximize the benefits of TRT.

---

163   http://www.trtrev.com/get-serious

CALORIC INTAKE IS DEPENDENT ON ONE'S GOAL

Your total food (macronutrients-protein, carbohydrates and fats) intake is always dependant on your overall goal.

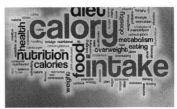

There are 3 distinct phases[164] or goals you can observe at any one time.

Goal	Caloric Consumption	Example
Maintenance of current body weight	14-16 calories per pound of total body weight in pounds	200-pound man would need 2,800-3,200 calories per day to maintain his present condition
Body fat loss	9-13 calories per pound of total body weight in pounds	200-pound man would need 1,800-2,300 calories per day to lose body fat
Lean muscle gain	17-20 calories per pound of body weight in pounds	200-pound man would need 3,400-4,000 calories per day to add muscle mass

You should understand how your specific body type (somatotype) processes and responds to insulin[165] when calculating your total calorie intake (respective of current goal). Insulin is the regulating hormone released by the pancreas when consuming carbohydrates. Depending on how insulin-sensitive you are, ultimately determines the amount of carbohydrates you can consume without depositing body fat.

As a man, it is important to familiarize yourself with your body type (somatotype).

---

164   http://fabfitover40.com/2014/01/01/tmcs-master-series-on-dieting-part-1-the-practical-approach/

165   http://fabfitover40.com/2014/05/21/managinginsulinforfatloss/

There are 3 different body types[166]:

- **Ectomorphic** (lean and skinny)
- **Mesomorphic** (naturally muscular)
- **Endomorphic** (heavier and higher body fat)

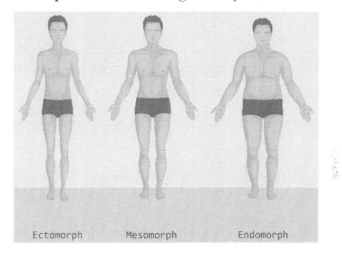

Ectomorph   Mesomorph   Endomorph

 TRT PRO TIP Most people are a combination of the 3 somatotypes. Those who are insulin-insensitive (endomorphic) will require a somewhat lower carbohydrate intake to avoid excess fat storage. This is why it is imperative to experiment on yourself with regard to your calorie intake and keep close records to see what works. All of the estimated calorie intakes listed above in the chart are highly variant due to biochemical individuality with regard to a person's insulin sensitivity. If you have higher body fat levels and are looking for a solution to strip fat off fast and as efficiently as possible, consider **Intermittent Fasting (IF)**[167].

---

166   http://fabfitover40.com/2014/05/23/howtohavecarbs/

167   http://fabfitover40.com/2014/11/28/interview-dennis-mangan-roguehealthandfit-ness-com/

THE SPECIFIC MACRONUTRIENTS NEEDED BY A TRT-ER

PROTEIN

Protein is made up of amino acids which are the building blocks of life. You need protein in order to build and maintain muscle. Protein is the most important macronutrient for performance and physique improvement. A protein rich diet is essential for optimizing 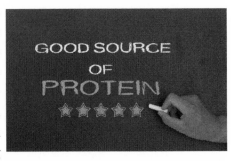 body composition whether your goal is fat loss or muscle gain.

Your daily protein requirements are based on your goals. Studies indicate an intake of ***0.7 to 1 gram of protein per pound of body weight*** is required to support the anabolic (tissue building) processes in weight lifters[168]. When undergoing testosterone replacement therapy, it is essential to always try and consume **at least 1 gram of protein per pound of bodyweight** no matter your goal.

 If you're worried that consuming high levels of protein might be detrimental to your kidneys, rest easy. The myth that high protein diets impair kidney function is based on studies carried out on those with renal disease. In otherwise healthy individuals protein intakes well in excess of one gram per pound of bodyweight have shown no adverse effects on kidney function[169],[170]. As long as you don't have any pre-existing kidney disease, a higher protein diet should pose no issues to your health.

To better understand the role protein plays in human nutrition, and the optimal types of protein to eat, read the following articles: Protein

---

168   Campbell B, Kreider RB et al. International Society of Sports Nutrition position stand: protein and exercise. J Int Soc Sports Nutr. 2007; 4:8

169   Martin WF, Armstrong LE, Rodriguez NR, Dietary protein intake and rental function. Nutr Metab(Lond) 2005; 2:25

170   Poortmans JR, Dellalieux O. Do regular high protein diets have potential health risks on kidney function in athletes? Int J Sport Nutr & Exerc Metab. 2000; 10(1):28-38

for Dummies Part I[171], Protein for Dummies Part II[172], and Protein for Dummies Part III[173].

CARBOHYDRATES

There continues to be dietary confusion that carbs are inherently detrimental to body composition. As such, many men have a form of 'carbophobia' and consume too few carbohydrates. Always think of your carb consumption as *time specific* and *goal dependent.*

Whether your goal is to *maintain your current body weight, lose body fat* or *increase muscle mass*, harnessing the power of your body's insulin production[174] is critical. The best way to do this is through carb cycling. For the optimal carbohydrate food sources to consume, there are the carbs you should eat[175].

To keep it simple let's analyze it based on 2 of the specific goals already discussed.

MUSCLE GAIN:

You'll consume between *1.25 to 2 grams of carbs per pound of bodyweight.* For example if a man weighs 200 pounds, then he will eat 250-400 grams of carbs per day to put on muscle weight.

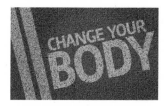

FAT LOSS:

You'll consume between *0.15 and 0.50 grams of carbs per pound of bodyweight.* (This is an estimate only and every person is different due to varying biochemical individuality.) Using a 200-pound man as an example, he should eat 30-100 grams of carbs per day to lose body fat. The higher your body fat, the less carbs you will consume. Again make sure your carbs come from the right sources[176].

---

171   http://fabfitover40.com/2014/02/25/protein-dummies-part/

172   http://fabfitover40.com/2014/02/27/protein-dummies-part-ii/

173   http://fabfitover40.com/2014/03/03/protein-dummies-part-iii/

174   http://fabfitover40.com/2014/05/21/managinginsulinforfatloss/

175   http://fabfitover40.com/2014/04/18/carbs-you-should-eat-2/

176   http://fabfitover40.com/2014/04/18/carbs-you-should-eat-2/

From a muscle building standpoint, most men seem to do best consuming *2 grams of carbs per pound of bodyweight*. For endomorphic men (usually insulin insensitive) it is likely you'll have to consume much less. As continually advised throughout this book, it is critical to establish BASELINES and self-experiment to figure out how your body type individually responds to your carb intake.

FATS (ESSENTIAL FATTY ACIDS)

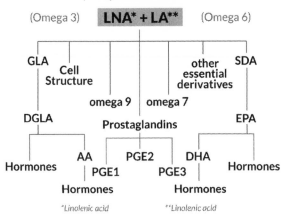

ESSENTIAL FATTY ACIDS
Critical Parent Components
for many body functions and structures

(Omega 3) **LNA* + LA**** (Omega 6)

GLA
Cell Structure
other essential derivatives   SDA

omega 9   omega 7

DGLA
Prostaglandins
EPA

Hormones
AA   PGE2   DHA
Hormones
PGE1   PGE3

Hormones   Hormones

Linolenic acid   **Linolenic acid

There is no more important nutrient to the human body than Essential Fatty Acids – commonly referred to as EFA's. Without them, your brain would stop functioning and your nervous system would shut down. They are involved in cushioning your internal organs for protection, aiding in the absorption of vitamins and minerals, and facilitating the production of hormones and prostaglandins.

Their consumption greatly impacts testosterone levels. Unfortunately *90% of people are EFA deficient* from eating a "normal everyday diet." Yes, you read that correctly. A diet high in essential fatty acids will help to keep your body in a state of positive nitrogen retention (anabolic) ensuring your TRT is maximally optimized.

How do you get them in your daily diet? And how do you best maximize their usage to improve your health and fitness? The only way they can be obtained is through select food and nutritional supplements.

I recommend getting them in these specific ways:

- Omega 3 Fatty Acids[177] (3-5 grams daily from pharmaceutical grade fish oil capsules)
- Coconut Oil[178] (2-3 tablespoons daily when cooking)
- Wild Cold Water Caught Salmon-Cod and/or Sushi consumption (1-2 servings a week)
- Red Palm Oil[179] (2-5 grams daily from capsules or 1-2 tablespoons daily from Pure Red Palm Oil[180] added when cooking)

SUPPLEMENTATION TO MAXIMIZE TRT

It is important to realize highly active and intense training individuals need adequate vitamin and mineral replenishment. Dr. Brett Osborn has a full list of supplements[181] he recommends in GET SERIOUS and I'm also providing a quick hitter list of essential things I believe a practicing TRT-er should add to their nutritional regimen.

Eating broccoli, cauliflower and cabbage will help rid the body of excess estrogen[182].

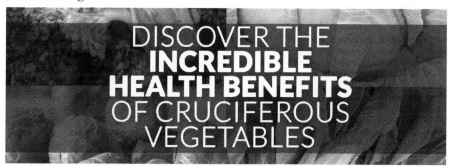

DISCOVER THE **INCREDIBLE HEALTH BENEFITS** OF CRUCIFEROUS VEGETABLES

---

177   http://trtrev.com/omega-3

178   http://trtrev.com/coconut

179   http://trtrev.com/red-palm

180   http://trtrev.com/pure-red

181   http://www.fabfitover40.com/supplements

182   http://fabfitover40.com/2014/01/14/is-alcohol-in-moderation-really-good-for-you-2/

You should already know by now why reducing estrogen is important. Cruciferous vegetables are high in **indole-3-carbinol** which is an estrogen-lowering food compound.[183] These veggies are also high in fiber[184] which help with weight control and body fat loss[185].

The body uses *Magnesium* and *Zinc* to maintain normal nerve and muscle function. Both minerals also support a healthy immune system, keep the heartbeat steady, and help bones remain strong. *Magnesium* and *Zinc* can also significantly increase free testosterone levels in men.[186]

Calcium hydroxyapatite improves bone mineral density and strengthens ligaments and tendons at the same time. All 3 of these minerals are found in the supplement Ultra Bone-Up. I highly recommend its usage when undergoing intense and heavy resistance training (**3 capsules twice a day** taken with meals).

It is also recommended you supplement with **Curcumin**[187] which is a potent antioxidant. Curcumin was recently found to decrease oxidative stress responsible for suppressing testosterone production in aging males[188]. **Curcumin** is one of nature's super nutrients and a powerful ally in the protection against cancer and in assisting healthy aging. It is also a powerful nutrient in fighting arthritis. **500 mgs 3-5x a day** with food is an optimal dosage and essential to protect and strengthen joints and soft tissues during bouts of heavy resistance training.

Ubiquinol Kaneka QH Coenzyme Q-10 (CoQ-10)[189] is a vitamin-like substance found throughout the body, but especially in the heart, liver, kidney, and pancreas. Coenzyme Q10 may protect against many age-related disorders, including cancer, heart disease, diabetes, and

---

183   Indole-3-carbinol, a vegetable phytochemical, inhibits adipogenesis by regulating cell cycle and AMPKα signaling. Biochimie. 2014 Sep;104:127-36. Epub 2014 Jun 18.

184   http://fabfitover40.com/2014/05/12/the-importance-of-fiber-in-your-diet-2/

185   http://fabfitover40.com/2014/06/23/fab-fit-40s-review-vpx-meltdown-2-holy-grail-fat-burners/

186   Effects of magnesium supplementation on testosterone levels of athletes and sedentary subjects at rest and after exhaustion. Biol Trace Elem Res. 2011 Apr. Epub 2010 Mar 30.

187   http://www.trtrev.com/curcumin

188   Abarikwu SO, Akiri OF et al. Combined administration of curcumin and gallic acid inhibits gallic acid-induced suppression of steroidogenesis, sperm output, antioxidant defenses and inflammatory responsive genes. J Steroid Biochem Mol Biol 2014;143, 49060

189   http://trtrev.com/q10

various neurological disorders. Supplementing with it at **200-300 mgs a day** is clinically proven to offer powerful anti-aging benefits[190].

Resveratrol[191] is a compound found in the skins of red grapes. It is a potent antioxidant and especially important in helping prevent the premature aging of your cells[192]. Supplementing at **100-250 mgs a day** is a proven anti-aging strategy.

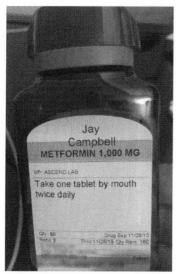

Metformin[193] is a powerful blood sugar regulating medication. Metformin increases one's insulin sensitivity[194] and by virtue, lowers circulating levels of the inflammatory hormone insulin. Having less inflammation will lead to a longer life. Between **500 mgs to 1 gram AM and PM** provides a wide range of therapeutic benefits including enhanced fat loss when used with a reduced calorie diet. In order to use Metformin, you MUST have a script from your doctor.

As previously written in Chapter 9, it is rare clinical doses of TRT can put undue stress on the liver. It is important to understand men living in large population centers are under continual bombardment by a host of toxins like phytoestrogens from the air, plastics and processed food. Most people consume excess alcohol as well. Even if you just recreationally drink alcohol, detoxifying your metabolic system via a powerful liver protectant is a good protective policy. I recommend Tyler Liver Detox[195] as an excellent overall detoxification supplement.

As shown in Chapter 9, the prostate risks are overstated when on clinical dosing protocols of TRT. Your physician can also prescribe

190   Dhanasekaran M, Ren J. The emerging role of coenzyme Q-10 in aging, neurodegeneration, cardiovascular disease, cancer and diabetes mellitus. Curr Neurovasc Res. 2005 Dec;2(5):447-59.

191   http://trtrev.com/resveratrol

192   http://trtrev.com/defy-resveratrol

193   http://fabfitover40.com/2014/12/28/life-extension-bottle-use-metformin/

194   http://fabfitover40.com/2014/05/19/eating-low-carbs-lowers-training-intensity/

195   http://trtrev.com/tyler

precise and effective BPH medications when necessary. I believe it prudent to cover all your bases with one of the strongest over the counter (OTC) supplements on the market today – New Chapter Prostate 5LX[196].

WHAT TO MINIMIZE AND AVOID WHILE ON TRT

Even alcohol in moderation[197] will lessen the effects of TRT. Alcohol increases estrogen conversion which is a big no-no for the many reasons already discussed. It also puts undue stress on the liver. Alcohol also has direct toxic effects on the testes and dramatically decreases testosterone[198]. I understand telling men to give up alcohol will be met with great resistance. I can't tell you what to do but I can damn sure tell you how to optimize your TRT protocol. If you want the best experience while on TRT, minimize your alcohol consumption.

After consuming sugar, testosterone levels decrease due to the release of insulin from the pancreas.[199] The human body rarely needs sugar. The rare exception is simple sugars immediately after an intense weight training session[200]. Other than consuming immediately post-workout—eating simple sugars including refined and processed carbs should be avoided as much as possible. You should also limit your consumption of NCAS (non-caloric artificial sweeteners) a.k.a. sugar substitutes as they have been linked to obesity[201].

196   http://trtrev.com/new-chapter

197   http://suppversity.blogspot.de/2014/06/true-or-false-occasional-weekend.html

198   Rachdaoui N, Sarkar DK. Effects of Alcohol on the Endocrine System.Endocrinology and metabolism clinics of North America 2013;42(3):593-615. doi:10.1016/j.ecl.2013.05.008.

199   Aromatase, adiposity, aging and disease. The hypogonadal-metabolic-atherogenic-disease and aging connection Cohen, P.G. Medical Hypotheses , Volume 56 , Issue 6 , 702 – 708

200   http://fabfitover40.com/2014/04/25/the-1-rule-for-building-a-fabulously-fit-body/

201   Sanz Y, Santacruz A, et al. Gut Microbiotain obesity and metabolic disorders. Proc Nutr Soc 2010:69:434-41

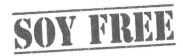

Consuming soy protein and its various friends[202] are absolutely counterproductive to maximizing TRT. As already pointed out, male endocrine systems are being bombarded by a host of environmental factors causing breast enlargement (gynecomastia), decreased facial and body hair growth, decreased libido, mood swings, higher body fat deposition, erectile dysfunction, and lowered sperm count. That is a brutal list and you would be wise to avoid soy protein and soy protein by-products as much as possible. So many processed and refined foods have soy by-products in them, you have to be supremely cautious and an astute label-reader to prevent its consumption.

Proper Hydration-How Much Water is Enough?

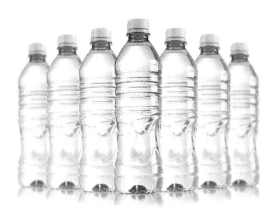

Water is the principal component of plasma and aids in the shuttling of nutrients through the bloodstream. It also aids in regulating body temperature, moistens the air for breathing and keeps our mucous membranes hydrated.

Water is crucially important to our body's two organ systems: the kidneys and lower GI tract. Both function almost exclusively to ensure excess water is not lost. It should be apparent drinking enough water will ensure proper metabolic functioning. You can also make it fun and

---

202   http://fabfitover40.com/2014/06/06/soy-protein-friend-foe/

rewarding[203]. How hard is it to drink 6-8 small 17-ounce water bottles a day? Apparently much harder than it seems for most folks. DRINK WATER. A LOT of it!

I highly encourage you to avoid or at least minimize consumption of carbonated beverages. The carbonic and phosphoric acid in sodas is horrible on your digestive tract and is a chief component of metabolic syndrome.[204] It also wreaks havoc on your gums and tooth enamel[205].

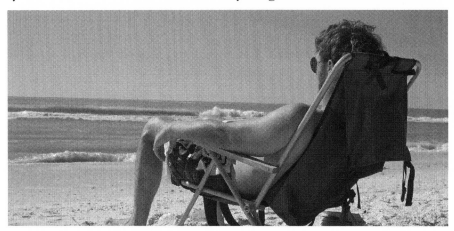

THE IMPORTANCE OF VITAMIN D FROM SUNLIGHT AND SUPPLEMENTATION

Yes you heard that right. Get out in the sun for 10-20 minutes 3-4 days per week or visit a tanning salon that offers beds minimizing/avoiding harmful UV spectrum rays. I AM NOT ADVOCATING sitting in a tanning bed and receiving a fake bake. I am saying you need sunlight and in areas where there is minimal daily sunlight, you need to come up with a workaround. Vitamin D is CRUCIAL to the formation of the sperm cells[206] and to the production of natural and free

---

203   http://fabfitover40.com/2014/10/22/get-drink-water-need/

204   The Oslo health study: soft drink intake is associated with the metabolic syndrome Appl Physiol Nutr Metab.2010 Oct;35(5):635-42.doi:10.1139/H10-059.

205   Effect of soft drinks on the release of calcium from enamel surfaces.Southeast Asian J Trop Med Public Health. 2013 Sep;44(5):927-30

206   Vitamin D and male reproduction. Nat Rev Endocrinol. 2014 Mar;10(3) Epub 2014 Jan 14.

testosterone.[207] Its supplementation is also significantly associated with total testosterone and SHBG[208].

To make sure you get enough (not being able to fully control how much sunlight exposure you'll receive) I recommend you have your physician test your blood levels of **Vitamin D, 25-Hydroxy** to make sure you fall into the upper end of the accepted value range of **30-100**. To ensure your score is *70 or above*[209], I recommend supplementing **5,000-10,000 iu's of Vitamin D**[210] **daily.**

Vitamin D is the name given to a vitally important group of micro-nutrients. When activated, vitamin D becomes a potent steroid hormone, switching our genes on or off, and instructing our cells what work to do. Vitamin D's effects are varied and profound. It is structurally similar to steroids such as testosterone, cholesterol, and cortisol (though vitamin D3 itself is a secosteroid). In other words, it's more of a hormone than it is a vitamin. Since too much vitamin D can become toxic, I recommend checking your D3 levels with a simple blood test.

---

207   Vitamin D levels and bone mineral density: are LH levels involved in the pathogenesis of bone impairment in hypogonadal men? J Endocrinol Invest. 2014 Oct 17

208   Vitamin D is significantly associated with total testosterone and sex hormone-binding globulin in Malaysian men Kok-Yong Chin, Soelaiman Ima-Nirwana, Wan Zurinah Wan Ngah
(doi: 10.3109/13685538.2015.1034686)

209   Andrology. 2014 Sep;2(5):748-54. doi: 10.1111/j.2047-2927.2014.00247.x. Epub 2014 Jul 16.

210   http://trtrev.com/vitamin-d

CHAPTER 11 READER QUESTIONS

What do you think of injectable nutrients? Do they work? What should be avoided?

Injectable nutrients are another way to optimize your supplementation. Some nutrients cannot be orally ingested due to mal-absorption or simply because high levels of nutrients cannot be obtained when digested orally. When injected, many nutrients can have a potent and direct effect which can be beneficial to performance or for the treatment of certain conditions.

Injectable nutrients can be hard to obtain since they require a prescription and are only available through specialized pharmacies, but there are progressive clinics that can offer them and have the medication shipped directly to you: http://trtrev.com/nutrient-injections

TRT AND FITNESS

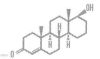

CHAPTER 12

THE FOUNDATIONAL ROLE OF WEIGHT TRAINING

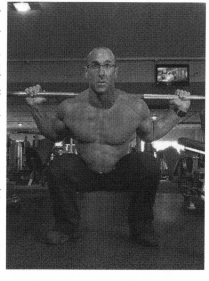

This book was not written to discuss the science and varying modalities of modern day weight training. This chapter offers a very high level summary of the influence resistance (strength) training SHOULD play in maximizing the success of testosterone replacement therapy.

Using testosterone and not performing regular weight training along with consistent endurance work (otherwise known as cardiovascular exercise) is akin to driving a Ferrari and putting water in the gas tank. Remember men, we're only as old as our arteries.

TRT enhances your body's ability to improve protein synthesis[211], increasing lean muscle tissue and reducing body fat[212]. Not taking advantage of its potent anabolic effects is counterproductive and pointless. Regular endurance exercise also exerts protective effects on

---

211   Anabolic applications of androgens for functional limitations associated with aging and chronic illness. Bhasin S1, Storer TW. Front Horm Res. 2009;

212   Testosterone as potential effective therapy in treatment of obesity in men with testosterone deficiency: a review. Saad F1, Aversa A, Isidori AM, Gooren LJ. Curr Diabetes Rev. 2012 Mar;8(2):131-43

the vascular system[213] including nitric oxide release, LDL quantities, and reduction of serum inflammatory markers. The last thing you want to be is a muscular individual who gets winded walking up a flight of stairs.

It is important to remember testosterone is only an adjunct to a healthy lifestyle. It's not a magic bullet nor is it exercise in a bottle. To maximize your hormonal response from TRT, train intensely with weights and perform low-impact endurance exercise. Repeat that again and learn to make weight training and endurance exercise a regular part of your life while undergoing TRT.

BUILDING MUSCLE AND STRENGTH

It is imperative for men to weight train large muscle groups with foundational strength exercises with planned progression: **Squat, Overhead Press, Bench Press, Deadlift and Pull Ups are optimal weight lifting exercises for men using TRT. 2x-4x per week for 45 minutes to 60 minutes per session** (depending on if training alone or with a partner).

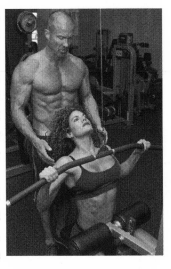

Utilize these principles in an optimal workout program[214]. This workout program is elaborately explained in GET SERIOUS. As already stated, I recommend you purchase that book.

You must learn how to maximally contract muscle fibers[215] by improving your 'mind-muscle connection[216]'. The more you can improve this communication/signaling between your mind and your muscle

---

213   Moderate cardiorespiratory fitness is positively associated with resting metabolic rate in young adults. Mayo Clin Proc. 2014 Jun;89(6):763-71.Epub 2014 May 5.

214   http://fabfitover40.com/current-workout/

215   http://fabfitover40.com/2014/05/09/do-you-know-how-to-maximally-contract-your-muscle-fibers/

216   http://www.t-nation.com/training/mind-muscle-connection-fact-or-bs

fibers, the more muscle fibers you will be able to contract leading to a much improved physique.

You can utilize various intensity techniques like Rest Pause Training[217], Supersets, varying rest intervals between sets and 4 Second Eccentrics[218]. Mastering these techniques is the quickest way to build muscle mass as efficiently as possible.

You must eliminate ego and momentum[219] from your training through controlled cadence (rep speed) and strict lifting form and technique. If you don't understand how to train with weights using proper form and technique, consider investing in a quality personal trainer or coming to **S.O.A.R.**: http://trtrev.com/soar

THE CARDIO EQUATION-HOW MUCH AND WHAT KIND?

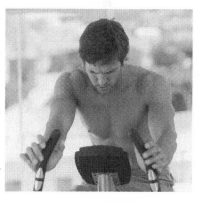

It is the author's opinion an optimal strategy for cardiovascular training is to perform *low-impact endurance exercise 2-5x per week* depending on body fat levels.

Optimal forms include *walking outside*, *walking on a treadmill on an incline*, a *stationary bike*, a *StairMaster*, *rowing machine* (ergometer) an *elliptical* or even *swimming*. As long as you take care of your soft tissues and avoid repetitive pounding on hard surfaces, your body will adapt well and you should be able to avoid injury.

If you have higher body fat and desire to lose it efficiently and quickly, you can up the intensity of your endurance exercise—possibly performing interval training[220].

---

217   http://fabfitover40.com/2014/09/15/ffover-40s-rest-pause-workout-explained/
218   http://fabfitover40.com/2014/07/23/want-high-thick-ridge-clavicular-pec-muscle/
219   http://fabfitover40.com/2014/08/01/ego-and-momentum/
220   http://fabfitover40.com/2014/04/23/12-steps-to-a-fabulously-fit-body/

It is CRITICALLY IMPERATIVE as an aging male you do not perform high impact endurance exercise (like running on hard surfaces, or ballistic movements such as those found in CrossFit programs etc.) in order to preserve your soft tissues and spine. The last thing you want is having your knee or hip replaced later in life because that type of activity can lead to life in a wheelchair[221].

The Importance of Sleep

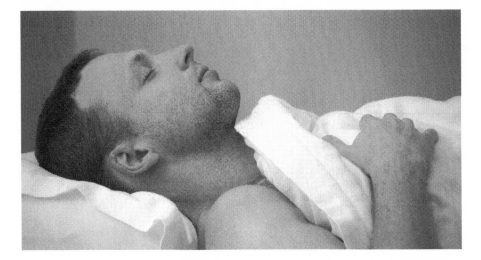

Recently, the critical *importance* of sleep has come to the forefront due to conclusive evidence for sleep's role in a variety of disease processes including obesity, coronary artery disease and neurodegenerative diseases such as Alzheimer's and dementia.

Adequate rest also can't be underestimated when it comes to optimizing recovery from the damage and stress applied to muscle fibers from intense resistance training. Sleeping with proper anatomical form[222] is also of crucial importance when it comes to avoiding stiffness and/or soreness to your neck and back.

---

221   http://fabfitover40.com/2014/10/10/running-and-cardio-can-lead-life-wheelchair/

222   http://www.livestrong.com/article/179141-correct-sleeping-posture/

Chapter 12 Reader Questions

Could you offer a Cheat Sheet or a Daily Dietary Schedule for a Man using TRT productively?

It really depends on what lifestyle goal you have at the current time. In other words, are you trying to **reduce body fat, maintain your present condition** or **gain muscle?** Here is a sample daily schedule for a Fat Loss Phase.

Fat Loss Phase

Wake Up – take 500 mgs-1 gram Metformin (rx from your doctor), Caffeine, Armour Thyroid 30-60 mgs (rx from your doctor), Thermogenic (MD2 is a good one[223]), Stinging Nettle Root[224] 1-2 capsules, inject your testosterone (if applicable for that day)

15-30 Minutes Later – 30-45 minutes of Low Impact Endurance Training (preferred types listed above) – aim for 70-75% of maximum heart rate (225 – age).

Meal/Feeding 1 – 30 minutes later 35-50 grams of protein powder[225], minimal carbs, 2 tablespoons of MCT Oil[226] or Udo's Oil[227]. Thermogenic 45-60 minutes later.

Meal/Feeding 2 (4 Hours Later) – 30-50 grams of animal protein, green veggies, oil dressing. Thermogenic 45-60 minutes later.

Meal/Feeding 3 (4 Hours Later) – Same as Meal 2.

Weight Training Day – Intra-workout shake with 25-50 grams of carbs and 25 grams protein (depending on your somatotype), followed by post-workout shake 30 grams of protein, 25-50 grams of carbs. If you are endomorphic (insulin sensitive) just use 25 grams carbs intra – and post-workout.

---

223   http://fabfitover40.com/2014/06/23/fab-fit-40s-review-vpx-meltdown-2-holy-grail-fat-burners/
224   http://trtrev.com/nettle
225   http://fabfitover40.com/2014/09/29/road-warriors-protein-powder/
226   http://trtrev.com/mct
227   http://trtrev.com/udo

Meal/Feeding 4 (Dinner) – Different form of protein (fish) and salad.

Meal/Feeding 5 (3 Hours before Bed) – 30-50 grams protein powder, MCT or Udo's Oil.

90 Minutes Before Bed – 500 mgs to 1 gram Metformin and 30-60 mgs of Armour. These medications will optimally work best in a low insulin environment (empty stomach) while you're sleeping at night.

NOTES

Individuals must have a Doctor provided script for Metformin and Armour Thyroid.

You will also have to assess your individual tolerance to the medications.

Set up caloric amounts based on what is already written above. Experiment on yourself and take notes always.

THE FUTURE IS NOW!

INTERVIEW WITH DR. BRETT OSBORN ON TRT

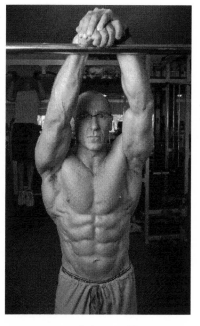

CHAPTER 13

Dr. Brett Osborn is a Board-Certified Neurosurgeon with certification in Anti-aging and Regenerative Medicine, a CSCS honorarium from the National Strength and Conditioning Association and over 30 years of exercise experience.

Dr. Osborn completed his 7-year residency at NYU Medical Center in 2003. He has performed well over 1,500 brain and complex spine operations. Also certified in Anti-Aging and Regenerative Medicine (by the American Academy of Anti-Aging Medicine), Dr. Osborn incorporates non-surgical modalities into his practice, emphasizing proper nutrition, hormonal optimization and strength training as preventive modalities. Practicing what he preaches, Dr. Osborn is the author of *GET SERIOUS, A Neurosurgeon's Guide to Optimal Health and Fitness* and co-founder of S.O.A.R. Seminars. Dr. Osborn resides in West Palm Beach, FL with his girlfriend Melissa Hankins. He is the father of three beautiful children: Jack, Ellis and Makenna.

JC: Thank you so much for doing this interview Dr. Osborn. Let's get right into it:

At this point in time very little consensus exists on 1) what constitutes low testosterone, 2) when testosterone supplementation makes sense, 3) what are the major risks patients face. From your anti-aging physician's point of view, how would you quickly answer or assess those 3 questions?

BO: Low testosterone is a clinical as opposed to a laboratory diagnosis. It is not simply "low testosterone" on blood testing. What constitutes "low" for one individual may be different than what is considered low for another. So-called "normal" testosterone constitutes levels that fall within a *huge* range. And herein lies the problem. You may have symptoms of hypogonadism (fatigue, loss of muscle mass, poor libido, etc.) and have T levels within the "normal" range. Likely you *would* benefit from testosterone replacement therapy regardless (provided other causative etiologies have been ruled out).

Unfortunately, most mainstream physicians fail to recognize that a "normal" T level means relatively little in the context of *symptomatic* hypogonadism. Again, what be considered a "normal" value (level), may not be normal for *you*. Discuss T supplementation with your doctor if you suffer from any of the aforementioned symptoms (which typically begin in one's early 30's). If he/she is unwilling to consider HRT, well find a new doctor.

The risks of testosterone treatment are minimal despite the media ranting. To date, not a single one of my *many* HRT patients has developed side effects from treatment. This is due to cautious prescribing habits. Side effects as discussed in the text include alopecia (low percentage of patients), prostatic "flare" (testosterone *does not* cause prostate cancer; this is a myth), polycythemia, low sperm count and in the case of injectable T, infection. These risks are far outweighed by the benefits of supplemental testosterone.

JC: It appears many doctors struggle with understanding the correlation between free testosterone and SHBG especially as men age. Do you have a preference between the free testosterone and total testosterone tests?

BO: Both free and total testosterone levels should be assayed. Why? The majority of circulating testosterone is protein bound. Albumin binds testosterone "reversibly." It has affinity for the molecule but freely releases into the tissues. Sex hormone-binding globulin has a higher affinity for testosterone (and other sex hormones) and binds them "irreversibly." Once bound therefore, it is unavailable to the tissues as SHBG does not readily release its grip on the molecule. That said, an SHBG level must be obtained as well. Noting all three levels, your physician will best be able to tailor your therapy. You may have high-normal Total T levels but very low Free T due to high levels of circulating SHBG (essentially gobbling up your manhood). This can be remedied easily with the addition of **stinging nettle root extract**[228] (and other agents potentially). Obtaining these values in isolation is worthless.

JC: **In the book I discuss how in my experience many endos/ doctors inaccurately dose injectable testosterone (cypionate/ enanthate) allowing for too many peaks and valleys creating a roller coaster effect of T and E. In your practice, how do you avoid this?**

BO: I use testosterone cypionate in my practice and dose according to my knowledge of its half-life. That said, I prescribe injections once or twice weekly (at half the dosage). *Patient feedback is paramount to optimize one's response to HRT.* If one feels better on twice weekly dosing, so be it. Levels of both T (total and free) and estradiol are checked frequently as to avoid any significant deviations from optimal levels. There tends to be a less aggressive approach in the community however. I know of many patients who were given prescriptions for T cyp injections once *monthly*. This carries with it significant risks, namely marked fluctuations in testosterone and estradiol levels in addition to dramatically stressing (and suppressing) the HPTA.

JC: **Let's talk about TRT and cardiovascular risk. How flawed are the JAMA and TOM studies?**

BO: Great question. And very timely. Simply put, the studies are flawed.

---

228   http://trtrev.com/nettle

There were several major flaws in the both:

1. **The men were not properly monitored and the dosages of T therefore were not restorative** (to levels offering previously demonstrated cardio-protection). The men enrolled in this study only boosted their mean total T to 332 ng/dL. This is low in the context of cardio-protection. See previous studies that such levels are associated with an increased risk of MI compared with levels above 500-550 ng/dL[229][230].

2. **Estrogen levels were not routinely assayed.** Likely many of the subjects aromatized T (testosterone) to E2 (estrogen) excessively, having not been placed on aromatase inhibitors (or similar medications). *Excess circulating estrogen predisposes individuals to thrombotic events.*

Bottom line, and likely for a variety of reasons, testosterone in physiologic doses (at optimal levels) is cardio-protective. How could the resultant increased vitality (and tendency to exercise which itself confers protection from cardiovascular disease), muscle mass and libido be associated with elevated risk of heart attack? Aren't these entities associated with youth? That said, adolescents exhibit very high levels of T on formal testing. When was the last time you heard of a 16-year-old male dying of a heart attack? Hmm, never.

JC: Is therapeutic phlebotomy a treatment for polycythemia? How many times a year should a man have his RBC's and hematocrit measured in his blood work?

BO: Many of my patients are routinely phlebotomized. I tolerate hematocrit levels of 50. Anything above warrants concern. I tend to be aggressive about phlebotomy to avoid any potential issues due to "sludging." That said, patients undergo laboratory testing at 3-month intervals initially. After optimizing their hormone levels, I will typically see patients (and obtain labs) every 6 months. In the interim, they are being phlebotomized per schedule (which ultimately depends upon their

---

229   Ohlsson C, Barrett-Connor E, Bhasin S, et al. High serum testosterone is associated with reduced risk of cardiovascular events in men

230   The MrOS (Osteoporotic Fractures in Men) study in Sweden. J Am Coll Cardiol. 2011 Oct 11;58(16): 1674-81

response to the prescribed blood draws: a STAT hematocrit is obtained prior to every phlebotomy session).

JC: **Do you believe patients with an elevated PSA but otherwise presenting in healthy/normal condition avoid TRT?**

BO: It is not unreasonable to utilize TRT in patients with elevated PSA provided the patient has a normal digital rectal exam (as documented by a urologist) and lacks urinary symptoms. I typically discuss these patients with the treating urologist who may opt to perform a biopsy prior to the initiation of TRT. Again, ***testosterone does not cause prostate cancer,*** but prostate cancer is hormone-responsive. Therefore, testosterone therapy should be avoided in individuals harboring *un*treated prostate cancer. A patient with *treated* prostate cancer however may be treated with the consent, and under the supervision of his urologist.

JC: **What's your strategy for the concomitant administration of erectile dysfunction medications specifically Cialis, Viagra, and Levitra while using TRT?**

BO: I have limited experience with these medications but have on occasion prescribed them. Of course, should there be underlying vascular disease (of which erectile dysfunction is often a harbinger), it warrants concern and mandates treatment. Phosphodiesterase inhibitors and the likes should not be used as a "workaround" for small vessel atherosclerotic disease. Again, this is about health. Erectile dysfunction is a warning sign, period.

JC: **Let's discuss the disease of aging and how it relates to low testosterone. Ronald Swerdloff UCLA MD and the co-author of the Endocrine Society's current Testosterone Treatment Guidelines recommends "measurement of testosterone on two separate occasions as well a thorough evaluation to look for chronic conditions, such as type 2 diabetes, that can lead to low T." What is your take on aging and low testosterone?**

BO: Chicken or the egg controversy reiterated. At this point, we as scientists are unsure whether hormonal decline "causes" aging or whether the converse is true. Regardless, as posed in the question, there are environmental factors to which the "disease" of aging (and age-related disease) may be attributed. In fact, there is indirect evidence that aging is 75-80% environmental in etiology. Keep in mind that "environment" encompasses ALL factors to which the body is exposed: nutrition, physical and psychological stressors and toxins to name a few. That said, many conditions such as type II diabetes and obesity, both of which have their underpinnings in insulin resistance, can <u>cause</u> hypogonadism.

The proverbial "quick fix" is to place a patient on restorative testosterone therapy, thereby correcting one's lab values. This however is a short-sighted approach, in essence addressing the epiphenomenon, as opposed to the phenomenon (type II diabetes in this case), or treating the effect and not the cause. I wholeheartedly agree with Dr. Swerdloff in this regard and routinely screen my patients for disease risk factors. In this context, I address BOTH the low testosterone AND said risk factors concomitantly. This is my practice paradigm. One is not addressed without the other.

Patients are started on a rigorous exercise program (as per the protocol outlined in GET SERIOUS), advised as to proper nutrition and supplementation, placed on medication (I utilize metformin, aspirin and antihypertensives aggressively) and counseled on the management of stress. Restorative hormonal therapy is often initiated concomitantly. The effects of the above are synergistic. Lowering disease risk factors (inflammation and insulin resistance) increases testosterone levels. Supplemental testosterone, in a reciprocal manner, reduces risk factors for disease. It's a double whammy.

JC: **With the FDA's recent ruling on adding Black Box Label Warnings to all testosterone products, is the landscape becoming better or worse for men seeking to optimize their hormones?**

BO: Neutral. I believe the FDA is simply looking out for the pharmaceutical industry and the populace at large. By virtue of their labeling, the FDA is exonerating itself as a governing body by indirectly publicizing the results, albeit flawed, of the recent TRT study. This should be held in the same regard as commercial-embedded warnings issued by pharmaceutical companies. And while attorneys may be chomping at the bit to vilify prescribing physicians in the wake of such labeling, this is by no means proof of danger (and likely is the opposite in fact). Answering your question, sometimes perceived "negative" publicity serves an antithetic function, and hopefully in this case will raise awareness of the health-promoting benefits of TRT in select individuals.

JC: **What changes do you see taking place on the testosterone front over the next five years?**

BO: The acceptance of TRT will continue to lag behind the robust manifestations of its life-changing effects. Millions of men and women are successfully utilizing TRT currently and regaining their vitality and lust (no pun intended) for life. And without side effects. Properly prescribed, TRT is perfectly safe. Its acceptance is simply a matter of its gaining momentum through documented treatment successes. A revolution of thought is in order. We are fast moving more towards a *preventive* health care paradigm and ultimately into one of *human* optimization. The treatment of disease post-facto will soon be of days yesteryear.

JC: **Talk about your practice—where is it going relative to all of the TRT clinics springing up across the country and the globe.**

BO: Continuing the thought my practice is currently a hybrid. The mainstay of my practice is neurosurgery albeit with a holistic slant. I make concerted efforts to treat all patients conservatively unless there are pressing neurologic issues which mandate surgery. Anti-inflammatory agents (high-dose omega-3 fatty acids and pharmaceuticals) are utilized as are exercise and nutritional strategies. Degenerative disease of the spine (affecting a large percentage of my patients) is an age-related disease. And herein lies the tie-in to Anti-Aging and Regenerative medicine. Treating degenerative disease of the spine is nearly identical to the treatment of all other degenerative diseases: coronary artery and cerebrovascular disease, diabetes and Alzheimer's dementia. It's just different geography. And *the aging process itself is a degenerative disease*, right?

This notion will drive the expansion of my practice ultimately. Many physicians have taken this leap of faith already, as the rewards (mostly financial) of primary care medicine have become virtually non-existent. And while it is unlikely that I will forego neurosurgery (patients will still fall ill), I plan on making every effort, through the looking glass of anti-aging physician, to alert the masses that we are simply doing it backwards.

JC: **Now that S.O.A.R. Seminars is out of the bag, can you provide your thoughts on who can benefit and why it's so unique in the current time and space regarding the improvement of HEALTH?**

BO: S.O.A.R. is GET SERIOUS personified. It is a multi-day seminar during which the individual is immersed in the concepts of Anti-Aging medicine. There are scientific, evidence-based lectures on the aging process, the role of hormone replacement (HRT), the foundational importance of mindset, and strength training/body mechanics in the context of safety and injury prevention. Patients will be thoroughly evaluated in a clinic setting and disease risk factors identified. These not only include metabolic and hormonal abnormalities as manifested in one's lab values, but one will also get a snapshot of his or her vascular anatomy (plaque burden) and cardiac function via ultrasound technology. Remember, "You are only as old as your arteries." The majority of us die a vascular death, right?

Aggressively attacking vascular risk factors therefore is critical. Insulin resistance and inflammation are BOTH dramatically improved through proper nutrition, exercise and hormone replacement (in select individuals). And this all begins with KNOWLEDGE. S.O.A.R. arms one with *that* knowledge, in essence empowering the individual and by virtue conferring longevity.

To learn more about S.O.A.R., visit this website:
http://TRTRev.com/soar

CONCLUSION

CHAPTER 14

When assessing modern day society, millions of men needlessly suffer from low sex drive, loss of energy, an inability to focus, soul crushing indecisiveness and a steadily diminishing enthusiasm for life—because of chronically low levels of their essential life blood—testosterone. Too many physicians who know little to nothing about TRT and even more lay people continue to be mystified by numerous misconceptions, both about testosterone's effects on human biology and behavior, and about the role of testosterone therapy in adults.

Testosterone replacement therapy is a verifiable and scientifically proven way to dramatically enhance your life. It should also be quite apparent "optimal levels" can be readily restored using the proven TRT protocols of progressive physicians.

It is important to thank the small number of dedicated physicians, scientists and active researchers who have devoted their lives to understanding testosterone's numerous effects on male life spans, and on building a factual, myth-destroying approach to TRT. This book is the result of close to 20 years of trial-and-error research, testing, refining, and a ton of blood (literally and figuratively), to deliver what I believe is THE authoritative research manual on testosterone replacement therapy.

My listed and recommended TRT protocols represent efficient strategies known to bring blood testosterone values to the highest end of the range while minimizing side effects and maintaining optimal health and safety. Rest assure, I and my research confidantes will be at the forefront of learning newer and more therapeutic protocols in the hopes of continuing the betterment of all men.

You should now be informed enough to speak intelligently with your TRT doctor. Together you should be able to formulate a plan for using TRT that will positively transform your life.

The ball is in your court to take action and optimize your Testosterone levels.

Remember, he who hesitates is lost (and likely the victim of low testosterone).

TRT RESOURCES

Even though it can be confusing sifting through the information found on the web about Testosterone, allow us to point you in the right direction to excellent websites, books and podcasts providing helpful information and answers to FAQ regarding TRT.

http://TRTRev.com/resources

Success Stories

Thank you for helping me change my life for the better! This week marks one year for me following your training, hormone and diet protocols. I appreciate everything you have done for me in my life."

Thanks again!

Matt

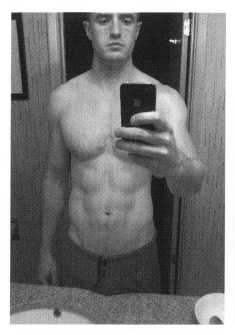 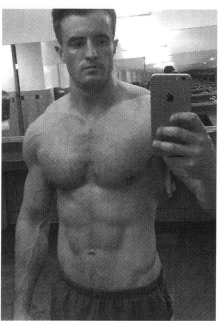

As a 48 year old man, and successful entrepreneur, I've taken my fair share of 'Test Boosters etc". I reached out to Jay and then began a program with him for about 4 months. I started out at 12% body fat. We optimized my hormones (I started a TRT protocol of 210 mg per week average) and cleaned up my diet. I used the workout regimen Jay recommends along with the medical advice and care of Dr. Brett Osborn. I experienced substantial increases in strength in the Squat, Bench Press, Overhead Press and Deadlift. The final two weeks of working with Jay, he prepared me for a photo shoot. I followed a specific diet plan and successfully dropped my bodyfat percentage to 5.5% and felt great with lots of energy! Jay's plan was 100% backed by science, and it worked exactly as he said it would!

Steve

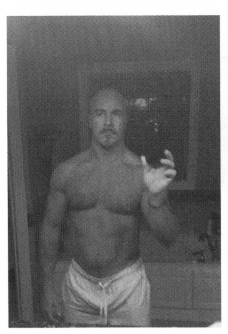
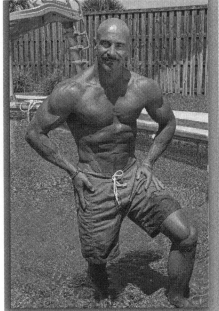

"Prior to working with Jay I was floundering in search of a new direction. As a 52 year old, I have put a lot of time in the gym but was in need of some fine tuning and a fresh start.

It isn't easy to find a levelheaded knowledgeable practitioner in the science of TRT!

Jay is a bold voice advocating a sensible approach in the context of health and longevity. Jay guided my protocol every step of the way. Jay would fine tune and refine my regimen both nutritionally and with regards to optimizing my TRT protocol but only when I needed it. The results have been spectacular."

Thanks for everything Jay

Tom

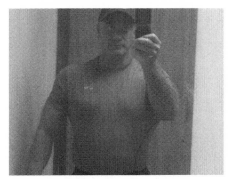
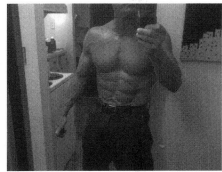

I started consulting with Jay close to a year ago. Although many people close to me would have considered me a successful person, behind closed doors I felt anything but. The energy I had felt in my early 20s was all but gone and here I was not even 30! I couldn't imagine what I was going to feel like by the time I reached middle age! I literally watched before my eyes as my social life, confidence, and muscle mass slowly but surely slipped away. Jay advised me on TRT and helped set up a consultation with a physician. Did you ever wonder what life would be like if you could go back to being 20, with the knowledge you have now? Well that's exactly what TRT allowed me to do!

With the proverbial eye of the tiger I attacked every area of my life that I had let slip by. With Jay mentoring me along the way I was able to not only put on 15lbs of muscle while losing fat, but transform my social and dating life to heights I had never achieved. With Jay's help I was able to get the excitement and energy back in my life that everyone should feel. He helped me realize I didn't have to just accept aging and there were logical steps I could take to combat it. With his help and guidance I'm now able to relive those younger years with the maturity of a healthy, hormonally optimal, 30 year old man.

Josh

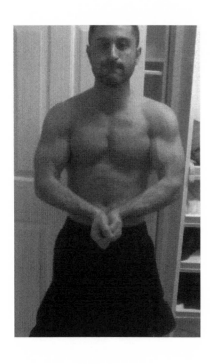 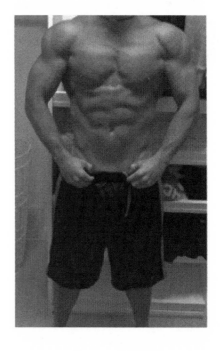

"Working with Jay Campbell and his recommended physicians has been a wonderful and life changing experience. As a relatively young former college athlete and successful sales professional, I never pictured myself as testosterone deficient. By following the protocol outlined in this book, I have gained twenty pounds of muscle, my libido is off the charts, and my nagging anxiety has been replaced with a steady, optimistic confidence. If you are a man who wants to go from good to better, or better to best, this is the book for you."

Jim N

NEXT STEPS

To Find a Progressive TRT Physician relative to your specific needs visit **TRTDoctors.com**

To consider signing up for the single most necessary and advanced 3 Day Age Reversal Conference on the planet, visit **SOARForever.com**.

If you WANT to take your Doctor-Prescribed TRT to the NEXT LEVEL, register for our Upcoming TRT Mastermind by visiting **TRTRevolution.com/Mastermind**.

ONE SMALL REQUEST

The information in this book can change the paradigm in the Men's Health Industry, and provide a real path to sustainable improvement in most aspects of men's lives. It can also prevent millions of men from suffering in silence from the debilitating effects of brain fog and depression.

In order for this book to reach as many people as possible, I'm depending on you! Please do me a huge favor and write an honest review. The more reviews it gets, the more this information will help others just like you escape from the conditions of sub-optimal Testosterone and transform their lives. I am sincerely grateful for the time and effort you put into writing a thoughtful review.

Thank you so much for reading *The Definitive Testosterone Replacement Therapy MANual*. I hope you use this information to transform your own life.

ABOUT THE AUTHOR

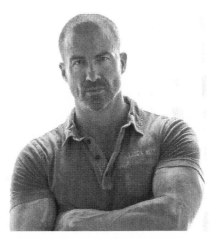

Jay Campbell is a champion male physique competitor and the co-founder of FabFitOver40.com-the number #1 site on the web for 'Fit over 40' information. Jay is also the Co-Founder of SOAR Seminars-a unique seminar that improves the aging process through optimizing biochemistry, utilizing the warrior mindset, and teaching proper strength training technique and mobility.

Jay is a 15 year Testosterone Replacement Therapy patient and recognized thought leader on Hormonal Optimization. Jay writes for Iron Man Magazine as one of the resident Anti-Aging Specialists. Along with wife Monica Diaz and Dr. Brett Osborn, they also produce a twice monthly webinar Health and Vitality Secrets for the Busy Professional, a live interactive forum for questions regarding Health, Fitness, Hormonal Optimization and Longevity.

Jay along with Nelson Vergel also hosts The Real Truth Men's Health Webcast - a monthly interactive discussion designed to help men achieve optimal health, fitness and vitality. Jay consults with men and women of all ages looking to optimize their health, fitness and well-being. Jay lives in Southern California with his wife Monica Diaz and is the father to two beautiful girls, Alexandra and Gabriella and bonus dad to Monica's daughter Alana and son Evan.

Made in the USA
Middletown, DE
14 March 2019